^{s}(Age)

Age Backwards

A Medical Intuitive's Guide To Aging

By Ethan Borg, M.A.OM, L.Ac.

Published By
Ethan Borg, LLC.
1427 Monroe Ave, 2nd Floor
Rochester, NY 14618 U.S.A.

Printed in the United States of America.
ISBN #: 979-8-9928700-0-8
For additional copies of this book, please contact:

Ethan Borg, LLC.
1427 Monroe Ave, 2nd Floor
Rochester, NY 14618
U.S.A.
support@ethanborg.com
Phone: 01(585)455-2828

Table of Contents

Ass High And Stunned

It is 1992. I am 20 years old. I am naked on Venice Beach in the heart of night. Minutes earlier, I was sitting in a donut shop with college friends (from Harvey Mudd College – I am currently on exchange from Swarthmore College) filled with the kinds of untoward characters that congregate in after-hour establishments in Los Angeles a few miles from the beach. It is funny how sharp memories can be formed based on spur-of-the-moment decisions powered by a midnight surge of sugar. "We should skinny dip in the ocean," said a friend. As soon as it was said, it was obvious: this was our intended destiny.

I am pulling off my clothes like they are on fire and throwing them behind me as I charge down the sandy embankment. To hide from the shivering cold, I sprint into the sea breaze, which doesn't quite solve the problem and yet I don't care. I am running in a black night towards a dark void. I cannot see into the void or beyond it and nevertheless I am full throttle. I am a fast runner. My feet hit the icy water's edge. The Pacific current in November is in no way a warm embrace. I envision running into the water until I am chest deep and then sliding gracefully above my head, like a boss, despite the breathtaking chill. My friends are hooting and hollering They are ahead of me and I want to laugh with them together as murr-filled mer-men.

I am ankle deep at top speed. I do not account for the transition from damp sand into wet waves with undercurrents. I immediately lose purchase. I belly flop and face plant, ass high in ankle deep water. I lie prone, awkward, and stunned.

I believe there may be no greater metaphor for the aging process than this. This is where we start.

Aging. It doesn't have to be this way; but this is how it goes for most of us. We don't all have to face plant ass-high into the dark void of destiny for failure to adjust to the obvious circumstances around us.

Life comes with no great guidebooks and this is partially due to humans being easily cajoled, berated, or outright fleeced by corporate interests as we cross multiple, confusing biomes of life. At each stage, we are sold a bunch of expensive lies by "experts" as to what would make us happy – lies that serve shareholder interests more than our own. It should therefore come as no surprise that the "age-ed" part of the aging process has no great road map even today so far forward into human history. Instead, there are plenty of side effect-laden pills, a host of mobility-assist products, and plenty of "it's just aging" advice to poorly direct us. As it stands, most of us are fated to awkwardly lose purchase rather than slide gracefully into the void.

I am 25 years in, a quarter century, as a traditional Chinese medical practitioner and this is the best guidebook I can offer you to fill this gap as to how to age gracefully and comfortably. It comes with no great promises. For instance, you are going to eventually die. Let's just start off with that hard truth. The aging process has an end point. We live in a society that wants you to never think about this or absorb it. Instead, we are supposed to get old but never quite acknowledge the elephant in the room. We are going to die and that's okay. We never had to be born in the first place. Every moment has been bonus time. If we are lucky enough to age then die – thank goodness – compared to the alternative. But to age gracefully with the fewest possible aches and pains, the fewest possible infirmities, well, I think that is the ideal circumstance – and that is what I hope for you as a goal in writing this book.

My father-in-law regularly jokes that he would like to avoid the aging process and prefers to be brought back behind the barn with his shotgun instead. I hate it each and every time he makes this quip. But I would like to point out, he is making this joke at 83 years old and has already undergone numerous surgeries, has been catheterized multiple times due to prostate issues, and has needed multiple rounds of at-home rehabilitation and physical therapy just to keep up with normal acts of daily living. He walks now with a sizable limp as he hand surfs tables, chairs, and couches to remain upright. For years now, he has told the same jokes over and over again without irony. Which is to say, aging for most of us is like the proverbial living frog being cooked in slowly boiling water. It is happening all around us even now. Indignities abound. Avoiding even one such indignity is a blessing.

It would be ideal to read this book when you are in your mid thirties but unfortunately we don't even think about aging until we are already pretty old. Most people who pick up this tome will no doubt be more than twice that ideal age, having already encountered a smattering of ailments that are part and parcel with being in a human body that has crossed the rubicon into the silver years. No worries, you can start to employ the ideas in this book right away. Just know that holistic theory is not like Western medicine. You don't feel better after you take the first pill. The ideas here take months and often even sometimes years to bear fruit – and the older you are when you start, the longer the path. Furthermore, you start where you start in the body that you have. Everyone will experience the benefits of my s(age) advice differently as a consequence. These factoids should be self-evident but by way of professional integrity, they must be said. Nevertheless, I do believe anyone can make use of these ideas at any time in one's life process and reap important benefits. Whether you are twenty or ninety, now is likely the very best time for *you* to start aging better.

Aging According To The Chinese Medical Classics

To say there are no guidebooks is obviously not exactly right. People have been talking about aging since the beginning of time. In my tradition of classical Chinese medicine, the oldest surviving textbook, the *Yellow Emperor's Classic*, discusses the aging process in its first chapters. It talks about people called Sages (from which this book gets its name) who lived hundreds of years because they were superior at adapting to the ever changing energies around them. Perhaps most notably, such people floated above the emotional viscissitudes of life. By feeling no emotion too strongly, they kept their internal energies at peace. In Chinese medicine, we believe most diseases first stem from strong emotions and therefore to maintain emotional balance means fewer physiological complaints.

While I find the idea of adapting to the ever changing energies around us sublime, the idea of not being emotionally invested in life absolutely rubs me the wrong way. This is not to say the idea is wrong. I believe it. I believe people who maintain emotional neutrality may very well live longer lives than those of us who live in a world of robust *feels*. But as my father says of my great great grandmother Julie who lived to 107: *only the last 50 years were terrible.*

God made the world a manuscript and people's feelings are notes of music upon it. Together, they make a symphony. There are high notes and low notes. It is magnificent and it is art. So, yes, perhaps if you opt out of being an instrument in this concerto you may live longer, but what's the point? If you feel like tofu, you're probably tofu.

Which is to say, my goal is not to promote this idea of deadening the senses to live a longer life. Instead, let's be invested in the grandiosity of the experience but try to get through it as pleasantly as possible however many years we have. To underline the point, even those Sages who lived long long lives in a state of emotional tofu – well, even they aren't around anymore no matter how long they supposedly lived. If you want to live a long life, live at emotional neutral, says the Classics. But if you want to *LIVE*, then don't focus on the years, focus on the quality. My hope is that this book helps you enjoy higher quality in a body with fewer complaints. With that, I am saying this is not necessarily a book about living longer. It is a book about living hopefully with less suffering. I posit that as a more meaningful arc. You may disagree. If all you want to do is live longer as your only goal, I have helpful ideas here for you, too, but philosophically, we will simply have to agree to disagree.

I'm Not Normal; And People Seem To Know It

It is 2001, and I am a third year acupuncture student in my student clinic rotation at a community health clinic that serves a poor population in downtown Boston. I work with many patients but one in particular is an older lady with severe pulmonary edema, with tremendously swollen feet, ankles, and lower legs. I am not prepared for what is about to happen. I insert needles in the swollen tissue to activate important acupuncture points. The points on the lower leg start to weep. A clear fluid drips down the leg. It drips and drips and, frankly, it doesn't stop. The leg is very swollen with fluid. I have a sudden fear that perhaps the leg will simply never stop leaking fluid. It isn't blood, mind you. It is like tapping maple syrup. I am highly professional in my demeanor but internally, I am feeling a sense of swelling panic that perhaps I have created a serious problem. Fortunately, the leg stops weeping. Rarely have I had such an appreciative patient even decades later. The treatments provided such relief to her enduring discomforts. We are good buds throughout those weeks of service to that community. Every week, the same thing. Points needled, legs weep, (I swell with temporary panic), everything resolves (except her overall condition remains unchanged), and yet, nevertheless, my patient expresses immense appreciation.

I have shared that I am a practitioner of Chinese medicine, which is based on a theory that everything we experience as physical first starts as energy. Energy is the key to health and disease. In our model, we call this: "energy first." We have a complex way of determining which energies are out of balance and how to restore balance in order to heal people of the myriad symptoms of disease that afflict the human condition. Chinese medicine is a theory of health and disease and there are three main tools we use to apply this theory to restore health: Chinese herbal medicine, acupuncture, and medical Qi

Gong.

Chinese medicine has been around anywhere between 3000 to 6000 years. Strangely enough, a frozen man found in the Swiss Alps, far from China, known as Ötzi the Iceman who died 5300 years ago, had tattoos of energy channels on his body that are the same ones we utilize in Chinese medicine (not all of the "energy meridians" mind you, but tattoos of some of them along with their respective acupuncture points). This is to say, there are many mysteries remaining as to the history of classical medicine and its prevalence over the planet. Chinese medicine as we know it, however, found itself the primary medicine over a landmass of millions of hectares across every nation in Asia over the ensuing several millenia. It was the main and only medicine for tens of millions of people who met it at birth and used it their whole entire lives applying it at every single health crisis without exception. There was no alternative. It treated infectious organisms thousands of years before Pasteur even was a zygote in his mother's womb. And even today it has survived hundreds of years of competition with Western medicine. It has survived because it is powerful and robust. It also offers different insights into the body than is afforded by Western sciences.

Chinese herbal medicine is an erudite, academic application of Chinese medical theory where we combine multiple herbs together into what we call "formulas" in order to make major changes to people's health and well being. Formulas combine herbs that individually might be too powerful, but in combination ensures people are not harmed by any one herb while allowing us to maximize the health benefits inherent within each component. It also lets us hone the medicine to specific areas of the body for faster results.

Acupuncture is what most people think of when they think of Chinese medicine. It is the manipulation of channels of energy along the body that we call *meridians*, in order to effectuate change in the tissues around those energy pathways. Through careful diagnosis, we select the right points in the right combinations to ameliorate health complaints. Sometimes needles are inserted into the body and sometimes needles are just held touching the skin (we call these non-inserted needles "teishin"). There are sub-methodologies within acupuncture that include burning a specific herb at acupuncture points or on needles at acupuncture points – a technique called moxibustion – and also applying suction cups to areas of the body for therapeutic manipulation of tissues (ie. breaking up adhesions).

The last major pillar of Chinese medicine is called "medical Qi Gong." It is as old as the other two. You may be familiar with the words "Qi Gong" as the first martial art that was designed entirely around self-cultivation, promoting energy balance and subsequently good health. Different body poses move energy to different areas of the body and these poses in combination restore energetic balance and harmony head to toe, inside and out. Medical Qi Gong, the third big branch of Chinese medicine, is similar to Qi Gong, but in this case a practitioner moves the energy of a patient without touching the patient with the goal of energy cultivation and re-balancing in order to resolve symptoms of disease. This is not done with body positions but with the mind. It is a "woo woo" art. You can think of it as the much much much older version of its very distant cousin known as Reiki. It is arguably the original energy medicine, though I am sure old shaman spirits around the globe might take umbrage.

I went to the New England School of Acupuncture, the oldest acupuncture school in the United States where I learned the first two methodologies. I was and continue to be obsessed with Chinese medical theory, endlessly tossing its theories in my mind well into my third decade of practice. It was a moment of sudden revelation of how disparate pieces of Chinese medical theory clicked together with Feng Shui that taught me the third pillar of Chinese medicine, medical Qi Gong. I am a medical Qi Gong practitioner primarily – which means I diagnose and treat people without touching them. I treat patients anywhere from a foot away to as far away as the other side of the planet. I diagnose and treat across any distance. As a consequence, I am not just a "medical intuitive" – someone who diagnoses health issues from a distance – but a medical intuitive healer – one trained in a rich theory that goes back generations before Ötzi took his first unfortunate, shivering steps up his last mountside.

I have been a practitioner of Chinese medicine since 1999 and in private practice since 2002. I have been lucky to be very successful in a field where success can be elusive. In the ensuing 25 years, I have experienced tens of thousands of patient visits – full days, working with patients every 30 minutes at a breakneck speed in general practice (which means, over my career, I have worked with almost every common life challenge that might arise – and a good share of uncommon ones as well). I have worked with every age group over the years, but it is fair to say that my clients have tended to be in their 50s, 60s, 70s, and 80s more than other ages. Which is to say, I have held a keen eye on the aging process from day 1.

I also have insights that literally no other person on the planet can make because I am innovating within classical theory. I think that is a funny concept, but it is also true. I have a curiosity that is ever hungry. Every day I work towards solving healthcare puzzles, bridging the gap between modern ideas of anatomy and physiology with classical theory. I am a seeker trying to understand the "why" behind problems not just with a modern vocabulary but also with one that is almost as ancient as "healing" itself. To be fair, some answers have come easily while others have continued to evade me. This book is the fruit of a very strange and unexpected career in which I have been obsessed about the mechanics of the body and the energy that constructs it. As a consequence, this book is not chapters full of high faluten platitudes that are ultimately vacuous or endless stories about me and my successes that serve no greater role than to puff up my reputation as a downpayment for future business. Instead, this is a book full of specifics and details at a level that I hope will shock you. That is my promise and I intend to keep it.

Medical Caveat

I am 2 years old. I don't quite get bubbles. Do you blow out or suck in? I also don't quite get the plastic bubble ring. Wouldn't it be easier to just make the bubbles with my mouth? I am sucking in directly from the bubble juice container. I am now choking on, gagging, and coughing bubble goo all over. I look around and find my sisters and parents laughing at me. My cheeks flush and I start to cry. "We're not laughing at you, we're laughing with you," becomes a common refrain of my childhood. It always confuses me, because I am never laughing at those moments.

Though I am a licensed medical provider, I am not your medical provider. Though in this book I am sharing findings, I am not ascribing these to you. You are a unique human with your own unique anatomy, physiology, microbiome, and allergies. If you put into practice anything that I mention in these chapters, please know that you are doing so from a guy who once drank bubble goo thinking he could produce bubbles from his mouth. I present myself as a professional with a quarter century of experience, but deep down in my core, I'm that kid. You are therefore understanding that you are choosing to follow my advice by your own accord with all inherent risks assumed by you. You would be best served – and I encourage you, implore you even – to discuss these ideas first with a licensed practitioner working with you, who knows you inside and out, before you attempt them. Allow a licensed healthcare practitioner to be your thought partner with you. We all need thought partners – not because we alone are d.u.m.b – but because life is complex and bodies are complex and often two brains are twice as magnificent as one.

The one thing I do prescribe for you, however, is based on watching my own parents go through the aging process, and also based on my moments of childhood foppery. Laugh more and especially at your own expense as you age. There are assuredly serious moments in life, but also you do not have to be serious about life's challenges and indignities at every moment. Yes, you might wet your pants just as you are about to greet the wedding guests. You might poop when you sneeze one day. You might face plant in front of the congregation just as you might face plant skinny dipping in the sea. Seeing the humor in moments that make us even more human may just be the best medicine of all. This is no easy prescription. But if you can master it, I believe it will serve you well along the shorter, bumpier side of the journey.

Not Your Everyday Medical Intuitive Guide

It is 1985. I am in middle school. I am at least two decades from figuring out I have intuitive sensitivity. Nevertheless, I simply know what people's fears are. I have no idea how I know these things. I can just sense it clear as daylight. Someone a bit smarter or malevolent might have used this intuition to manipulate people to get more of what he or she wanted in life. Me? I do absolutely nothing with this knowledge. If it doesn't help me in sports, it isn't all that meaningful to me. And this skill is useless from across the tennis court. In due course, I completely forget this skill. It never returns, even after I become a medical intuitive. I am not a spiritual prodigy in my youth. I have no encounters with spiritual guides. I don't hear dead people – and that's a good thing – as that would have scared the ever lasting crap out of me as a sensitive young boy. I engage in no sudden healing encounters presaging my future. I am just an average kid fantasizing about winning Wimbledon, following the footsteps of my tennis hero with the same last name. He is the garage door. And he wins every point we play.

If you have been a ravenous consumer of medical intuitive prose, you would find that many intuitives spend a good chunk of their writings about their psychic gifts, their first encounters with energy healing, and perhaps their first encounters with their spiritual guides. There is an "ooh" and "ahh" side of this behind the curtain backstory. To be generous, you can say it is to build confidence in their skills – to "buy in" to the story. To be less generous, one might say it is to hide the two dimensional nature of the advice that fills the shorter chapters that follow – while at the same time building a brand that is good for business. That may sound judgmental or cruel. I apologize if that is the case. But the reality is that life is a cacophanous mess and all of the problems in the human condition will not fall at the feet of a single infectious organism or some spiritual contract that needs to be broken.

It therefore helps to have a foundation in something robust from which to build. I am very fortunate that I learned Chinese medicine before I became an intuitive. It has served me far more than anything else possibly could.

I also was very very lucky to have gotten what was likely Lyme disease in my late teens and then to suffer for seven years of chronic fatigue. Yes, "lucky." The suffering was endless, despairing torture, but it also was a gift I could not in any way appreciate at the time. Up until then, I was going to follow my father's footsteps into Western medicine. I certainly had the aptitude and the gift of a photographic memory. But this suffering completely upended my master plan. Ultimately, it changed my path from Western medicine to Eastern medicine, and it turned out Eastern medicine was and is my one true vocational love. As I said, I was very very lucky to have discovered my intuitive powers *after* building a foundation in a very robust healing art with such strong, deepest of deep roots, as it was a stepping stone into dealing with the true challenge of healing many people from many genetic springs with many emotional misadventures whose ailments and diseases each had different starting and end paths. This depth meant I would begin my career with depth provided by the wisdom of people smarter and more observant than me and, with these gifts in hand, I have had the opportunity to only go deeper. Inasmuch, I won't spend as much time on my backstory. I won't ignore my backstory but I also won't belabor it. I am not writing this book to build my practice; it is full. I am not writing this book to sell products I make or other services I provide. If you want to learn more about me, I will share. But not so much in the meat of this book. This book is about you and avoiding likely pitfalls in your aging process. Most of this book is about *you* and how *you* can stay a "you" for as long as possible with the fewest life complaints.

I am attracted to blond haired, blue eyed women of a certain short stature. Every person meeting this criteria gets special consideration. By 8th grade, I have started to focus on women named Jen. I simply know I am looking for a perfect-sized blue eyed, blond named Jen. I meet her on August 25th, 1990. She is 5'3". Her hair is only blond because it is bleached by the sun from playing soccer but in short order will turn brown. One day, she touches my back and I feel her energy. It is the first time I realize I can feel energy and that ***energy*** *matters to me. It's three decades later and we still cuddle like squirrels in a Winter's nest. A brief sense of her energy at age 18 and she becomes the singular focus of my romantic desires. It will take another decade and a half before energy itself becomes my singular vocational focus. And yet, it has already revealed its absolute importance.*

Back then, I intuitively knew what I wanted. Let's talk about what you intuitively and logically want now. I am going to put words into your mouth and if I am wrong, just straight up burn this book for warmth. Big stakes. Here it goes: You want a good life. A good life is not an endless life but one that is so interwoven in good experiences you might just think it resplendent with lightness and light. No small part of this is good health, as your body is the foundation of your experience and it is also a major determinant of your mood. I would say a good life feels real. This means it is not a singular line in a singular direction but has ebbs and flows, ups and downs, with bouquets of emotions. That said, a bouquet with predominant lightness is more desirable than one with too many dark notes. You want to feel good emotionally and physically. And you want to age that way, too.

I also surmise that you want a sense of movement especially towards growth, satiety, completeness, and thriving. That sounds good, doesn't it?

Yet as we move in the direction of achieving more and more of our goals, the body works against us. It develops pains that maybe before were rare or intermittent that over time switch to being more consistent and chronic. New colorful molluscs show up on the thinning skin as an outward reflection of changes happening internally.

Contemporaries go from rarely having major health events to regularly having gatherings that turn into "organ recitals." The fear of not having enough time "on planet" grows at each decade and it starts unexpectedly young. Honestly, it feels hard to thrive when increasingly one thinks about death and dying.

Correct me if I'm wrong, but perhaps you want to think less about death and dying and more about living no matter your age. You want to age with less pain and at the very least no new pains surprising you as "long term squatters." Let's say this is possible, where do you turn for hope? Do you follow medical advice from doctors who increasingly diagnose your issues as "normal aging" instead of solvable symptoms? Do you buy endless supplements being touted by the same people who touted the last expensive supplements that made no practical difference even if they somehow make you feel good? Do you take advice from your friends who are aging just as quickly if not quicker than you?

Maybe, just maybe, you take advice from someone completely outside your normal realm of influence – perhaps someone who comes from a medicine that is not decades old or centuries old but thousands of years old. And, as an aside, when was the last time you did something that did not seem to help more than a few times – let alone again and again for 3000 to 6000 years? Which is to say, perhaps an outsider's voice that has behind it thousands of years of experience might be worth a listen. No one says you have to do a single thing I recommend. But a listen won't hurt. Your goals are my goals and this book is not a hidden predation on your hard earned savings. Your goals are my goals and I only want you to achieve them because I am at my heart a healer and nothing means more to me than you living with less suffering. Period. I write as an extension of my work. I can only see so many patients in person. I write to help more people than the limits of time. And like everyone else, time is my most limiting factor.

Intuitive Non-"Intuitive" Advice: Exercise & Eat Veggies

It is the Summer of 1992 (I have not yet gone off to California for a semester). I realize Western medicine's solutions to what decades later I would self-diagnose as Lyme Disease was a complete disaster. This is a major crisis for me precisely because I am pre-med in college. I have seen cardiologists, urologists, asthma and allergy specialists, orthopedic surgeons, and my primary care physician within the last two years and after getting nowhere with their pharmaceutical friends, I receive again and again the dreaded diagnosis: "it's all in your head." I must have a very strong head as the symptoms are intolerable and only worsening, starting with a terrible case of Mononucleosis, leading to an enlarged prostate with sudden panic-inducing urinary urgency, a full stomach the second I start to eat anything, flu-like symptoms every weekend, joint pains all over but excruciating at my right shoulder, angst with depression, and the terrible weight of fatigue wrapped around me like a suffocating blanket.

I make a decision: if it is all in my head, I trust my head and no one else's to solve my problems. The doctors had their chance. I turn to vitamins and minerals – go through scores and scores of these, adding one at a time to see if any single supplement will move the dial even the tiniest little bit. GNC, the local vitamin retail chain, is my friend and the cashier seems to like me quite a bit, too. Vitamin A seems to help; beta carotene, too. I eat carrots – lot's and lot's of carrots. I eat so many carrots and take so much beta carotene, my skin literally turns orange. This is not an exaggeration. I am an orange man. But I feel the tiniest edge better so call it a win.

It should come as no surprise – which is also why I will not dwell on this too long – that eating nature's garden of minerals and vitamins is far superior to eating processed foods when it comes to living healthier with fewer physiological and emotional complaints. The

Standard American Diet, also known as SAD, is a known killer but is also a lesser known "quality of life" (as in, it hasn't yet killed you) torturer. Sure, you might die young, but you also won't enjoy the process. You have that going for you every time you eat a blueberry muffin for breakfast rather than just blueberries. Diabetes, poor circulation, and elevated inflammation all join the house party soon enough if invited and SAD has sent out the invitations already.

There are many culprits but none is worse than sugar. Hear me out. Please read passed the next line: White processed sugar is *poison*. We have to acknowledge that. But it also tastes really good. We have to acknowledge that too. I eat it. I eat plenty of it. I'm no saint. Many of us elect to have this poison to enjoy our culinary lives and I say that this is fine so long as you seek moderation and make good decisions around all other aspects of your diet. But know this. It *is* poison. And it is in most of today's processed food. It is perhaps the absolute worst thing in your diet. Period. White processed sugar: bad. Drop mic. And if you eat a lot of processed foods, you are eating far more of it than you realize.

As I said, I am no dietary saint. Definitely not. Plenty in my field have chosen a low or no sugar path. More power to them! Me? I eat some processed foods and occasional desserts while making sure every meal without exception contains natural colors in natural things with as much variance in color as possible. The more colors the better. Making rainbows out of meals is best. You should already know this because it is not new and it is not rocket science: eat better; live better. Veggies are what we mean when we say eat better. Natural proteins are also ideal – nuts, beans, natural fats (ie. olive oil or avocado oil), and a small amount of lean meats round out a healthy diet. Me? I also eat chips, make homemade banana bread, have an annual "Ice Cream In February" birthday party every year, and I love a gelato (or dare say, an affagato) now and again, and so on. I am not out to win the esteemed and also made up "garden champion" award. But I do have a few motivations: to leave the planet as good or better than I found it, to kill as few animals as possible for consumption – preferably those that don't fart too much methane, and to live a healthy life as long as that blessing is possible. As an aside, I do have one rule around meat sources: if they can play, I won't eat them (that's my own personal guiding light). Cows can play. True story. Chickens, not so much.

In Chinese medicine, people develop a problem we call "Blood Deficiency" when they don't eat enough vegetables. This is not to be confused with anemia, which is a Western medical diagnosis that does not correlate one-to-one with our traditional model of Blood Deficiency (ergo the capital "B" in Blood). There are a wide array of symptoms that can come with Blood Deficiency including achy ligaments and tendons, difficulty falling asleep, blurred vision, heightened anxiety, lack of patience, heart palpitations and more. A telltale sign of Blood Deficiency are pale lips and pale fingernails. If you notice these features on your own body, eat more vegetables and stat! Some people simply hate vegatables and these people always look pale because they are Blood Deficient. No doubt, this is the basis of many chronic complaints. If you don't eat enough veggies, you complain one way or another. So many problems stem from this, it is crazy.

In recent years, I have come to associate Chinese medical concepts around Blood Deficiency as being the equivalent of suffering from low electrolytes. For instance, Liver Blood Deficiency now associates in my mind with low magnesium. Heart Blood Deficiency associates with low potassium. And so on. This explains the vegetable connection – if you eat an abundance of things that grow in gardens, you consume bioflavanoids, electrolytes, microbiome, and other building blocks of cellular shazam. This also starts to tie together diet with health and disease. Eat veggies and you are more likely to fall asleep easier (magnesium L-threonate is correlated with better sleep, by way of example). Diet doesn't just matter when it comes to your health, it is one of the few things you have control over that you can tweak day-to-day to heal and thrive.

Western medicine is literally in the gutter around diet and disease. I won't say a lot of negative things about Western medicine in this book outside of what I have written thus far because Western medicine does plenty of good. It is not either/or for me. We are all in the healing profession doing our best. But wow has Western medicine completely and utterly failed its consumers by ignoring diet to such a tremendous degree. We all know SAD is a terrible diet that increases arteriosclerosis and raises blood pressure as well as blood sugar, and yet there is no marker in your CBC (Complete Blood Count) for how many donuts you eat a month versus how many grapefruit. You might say that

shows up in A1C, SED rate, or LDL cholesterol, but if it does, where's the follow up questions about how many foods do you eat that come out of a fryer versus a Farmer's Market – and where's the advocacy to eat rainbows? This is a big error of omission. Perhaps the biggest.
Which means the reader of this book is in the same boat as I was in 1992. Your mind has to solve how to age gracefully – not the minds of the professionals who diagnose and treat you. I therefore encourage you to do the research yourself and see where this assertion originates in the scientific literature: eating more vegetables gets you more miles on this road with enduring tread.

There is another missing physician conversation around the quality of your longevity – how much do you move your body and in what ways? Do you move every joint? Do you move against resistance beyond the resistance of your living room couch against your buttocks?

I have a basic tenet: "use it or lose it." I am talking about your body parts, and especially your bones and joints. Most people work sedentary desk jobs only to return home to sedentary streaming video nights. Your body is blessed with joints not always in obvious places such as between your sternum and ribs, along your vertebrae, your clavicle, scapula, and shoulders, even your sacrum and coccyx. You have joints all over but are you making sure to move all over? This is where cardio exercise really shines – it ensures that you move your joints. You are more likely to retain flexibility in your body as you age if you move your body not just regularly but as close to daily as humanly possible. At the very least: walk. At the very most: dance. Seems simple enough. (And I'm not kidding about dancing. There is hardly any athletics better than dancing for moving every single joint).

Studies have shown that weight bearing exercise is absolutely essential in maintaining bone mass as you age. I have a secret to share with you about this: I absolutely hate weight bearing exercise. But medicine is medicine. I work with weights once a week. Is this enough? Probably. I am not trying to sculpt my body – just trying to keep it. I have reached a level with my weights where it isn't easy or pleasant to do the exercises but I am not ramping up the resistance any more than necessary. I'll let the body builders build their bodies, I am just looking to do the bare minimum to keep my bones. Which means I still need to feel like I did a workout when I'm done. At least a small amount of sweat is necessary confirmation. If you aren't sweating, you aren't exercising. If you walk, walk until you sweat…or you aren't really walking, you're just in light motion. If you live in a humid location, you can't use the sweat heuristic, but you should understand the thought behind it. Your heart has to pump a bit stronger than normal.

In this book, I will talk more about bones and their absolute importance. Yes, bones are the foundation upon which other structural tissues brace – but their importance expands far beyond that. Bones are energetically the coldest tissue of the body and this serves many important functions from an "energy first" perspective. Which is to say, keeping my bones full and strong is a giant goal in my healthy aging strategy. Inasmuch, I am willing to do what I hate – free weights. And I do it only once a week because I hate it. If you enjoy it, up to three times a week might be right for you when the goal is to avoid osteopenia and osteoporosis, to avoid losing inches of height, and to avoid losing the most important material that makes up joints – our boneheads and their cartilage. Which also means exercise is the key to avoiding joint replacements involving surgeries, unpleasant surgery recoveries, plus painful PT exercises for weeks and months.

What are you supposed to do if you already have osteopenia and osteoporosis? You are supposed to do weight bearing exercises. Period. And eat right. Period. You just need to make sure you have a professional Personal Trainer helping you start out with weights and perhaps a nutritionist as well (at first) to make sure you don't break a bone on our journey to build more bone mass.

Key Takeaways:

- The foundation of aging well is eating fruits, vegetables, healthy fats, and healthy proteins. Eating natural rainbows will provide you with electrolytes, bioflavanoids, and will support your microbiome
- Use it or lose it when it comes to joints

- Cardio exercise and weight bearing exercises are both necessary to maintain bones and joints
- Medical professionals have abdicated the most important role in medicine – making sure you do the homework you might not necessarily enjoy – eating fibrous vegetables and moving your body

Self-Care Tools In This Book

I am a practitioner of Chinese medicine and an innovator in medical Qi Gong. As you can imagine, the tools of the trade for me are very different from what you can find at a grocery store in Kansas City or a pharmacy in Rome. Yet, I am writing a book that I hope will serve you not just with knowledge but with immediately employable self-care strategies.

As I said earlier, please discuss the tools and strategies I write about in this book with your trusted healthcare providers. They know you and they will have informed opinions about my self-care suggestions as they might be applied or shouldn't be applied to you, specifically. Why does this matter? Mainly it matters because the tools I focus on in the core of this book are ones I believe you can find all across the world without any access to Chinese medical practitioners and the unique toolsets we employ. I am therefore bridging the gap between what I know, what I know my patients have used for self-care, and the problems that need to be solved for you to live with the least amount of suffering as you age.

The tools I suggest in this book are therefore **not** my main operative methods with my own patients, but the best suggestions I have for you based on these factors. Would I use caprylic acid or oil of oregano to kill yeast with my patients? No, I would use medical Qi Gong. Would I use hyperbaric oxygen chambers to kill anaerobic pathogens? No, I would use medical Qi Gong. Would I work on cavities with hydroxyapetite crystal toothpaste? No, I would use medical Qi Gong. But unless you are a medical Qi Gong practitioner, you will need to use the tools available to you.

In a few cases, there are simply no supplements or medicines that can solve the issues I write about in this book outside of my work…yet. And I include them in this book because perhaps reading about them here will inspire someone to cultivate such tools once they see how important they are.

The Five Protocols For Aging Gracefully

It is 2016. My professor wife is on sabbatical and we have moved our two children to Valencia, Spain for the next 6 months. We live close to the Turia, a river that has been diverted and the many kilometers of its old bed has been converted into a wide, serpentine park. Every Friday, I ride a city bicycle from my home, through this gorgeous green theater to the far end, where the famous, futuristic buildings of Valencia blossom like alien flowers. I meander North through a few city streets and make my way to the playa, the beach, where I promptly sit myself at the cafe with a view of palm trees, the wide sandy jet, and then the luxurious blue of the Mediteranean. I eat a couple super tiny croissant and enjoy a sugary coffee as the sea breeze lazily washes into the open aired seating area. Next, I walk midway to the sea and then lie supine, often covering my face with my shirt so as not to be blinded. And I realize how lucky I am to have these moments. These moments are precious. And we all should live long enough to have them in as much bounty as we are able.

These are also moments when I am not in our apartment near the botanical gardens that smells like sewage when my heart throbs with deep depression, being so isolated in a land far from home. These are not the moments when my no pork and no seafood diet, when I need to eat before noon so that I can call my patients at home in the United States at a reasonable hour, when I am swimming in frustration that practically everything but the water is full of pork and seafood and practically every restaurant that might entertain my needs opens at 1pm.

There is a great polarity in my experience of those six months. The travel is insanely amazing. We visit Barcelona, Madrid, Toledo, Seville, Cordova, Malaga, Granada, and Portugal and every location stirs the heart with adventure and discovery. Meanwhile, I am writing no less than 5 curriculum books for my students when I am not treating patients long distance with medical Qi Gong. I am not on sabbatical. My days have so little space, I have no time to learn the local dialect,

Valenciano, leaving me a stranger in these lands. The highs are so incredibly high and the lows are as low as I have experienced in my adulthood. Meanwhile, I would never trade this experience in for any other.

But I learn. I better understand what I need so that the next time I am blessed with such an opportunity, should I be so lucky, I can trade more lows for more highs.

Not every religion believes this, but for many, this is our one life. And even for those who do believe in reincarnation, I think it is safe to say we all face our life's experience without receiving many "how-to" manuals. As a consequence, there are no "next times" in the aging process and for each of us, we have to do our best to get it right *this* time. There are no "Loading Checkpoints" (you gamers out there know what I am referring to) to restart a section of our lives at a previous point in history to do it better the next time. We tend to carry our mistakes forward like a cartoon butler carrying more and more bags until there is no butler just a mass of baggage heading to the guest room.

There is no way to turn the entire clock backwards, but I do believe we can turn parts of the clock back in time up until a point. I believe in reverse aging to a degree. The clock will once again start ticking, but we can sometimes use our fingers to move the hands of the clock a few ticks back here and there. Ergo, I introduce to you the Five Protocols for aging gracefully that are designed to be used both ad hoc (as in, "when you need it") and also according to a calendar that I have added near the end of this book. I considered placing this chapter by that calendar which would make a whole lot of sense for quick referencing back and forth, but I also refer to these protocols again and again ad nauseum in the remaining chapters, making their placement early in the book a helpful exercise. I recommend placing a paperclip on this chapter and also at the calendar so that you can effectively make them as quick to reference as if they were side-by-side.

The Five Protocols reflect that we live in a far more complex world than most want to admit. It is easier to say that we only have to worry about one problem in life and that if we organize around that issue, all of our needs are met. The reality, however, is that our planet was a microbiol soup for literally billions of years before we even were glint in the eyes of our first ancestors. Billions. The biodiversity on this planet is mind boggling. Mostly, it is invisible to the naked eye and yet life is teaming all around us with a rainforest we cannot easily perceive and yet we engage with every day in everything we do. Even the person on this planet with the weakest immune system (ie. the "Bubble Boy") has the most amazing immune system when you realize that from head to toe we have a boundary tissue that is designed to fend off this invisible microbial kingdom that arguably rules the planet. Our skin does a splendid job. We are touching creatures day and night (not that we want to think too much about it) moment-by-moment there is a great division between what is inside us and what is external. We have mucus membranes on the inside, playing a similar role in defending our boundaries. And we have armies of white blood cells that are policing every millimeter of our system day and night. Yes, we get sick…and perhaps seemingly frequently. But the entire enterprise that keeps organisms from making our bodies their homes is friggin' AMAZING. Until it isn't. And this "until" is a slippery slope, a subtle voyage from being prime to being slowly overrun by the reduction of our system's own efficiencies and also the constant persistent nature of a microscopic jungle all around us.

The first thing I want to say before we go any deeper is this: we are not alone. We have friends. We have a microbiome everywhere head to toe throughout our skin and every millimeter deeper. Friendly microscopic organisms defend our systems from foes just as much as our own white blood cells. We are fully integrated with microscopic life that is "Defending The Gates" as we say in Chinese medicine. If the outside world of infectious organisms is a jungle, we have sophisticated, curated gardens of microscopic life that we literally cannot live without. We even receive nutrients our own bodies cannot digest that we only absorb by the good graces of the symbiotes that make up our flora.

It is a very juvenile, but also in many ways a totally reasonable response to living in a jungle of microscopic predators to think we need to kill everything around us and live in sterile environments. But the great wisdom of this creation, is that we cannot actually do this and be complete. We need to embrace the organisms that serve us and that we serve. We gain vitality from these organisms. Without them, we would experience tremendous fatigue and even malnutrition.

And yet, within these protocols, I do not reference probiotics in any way as a vehicle for generating a healthy flora. Instead, I suggest eating fruits and vegetables, live in the world, be active, embrace friends and family, and be in community. These are much better ways to restore your microbiome right now. I say this because the microbiome is made up of hundreds of thousands of unique species and yet at our level of knowledge and technology, we only have access to perhaps up to 25 species that you might take in supplemental form. It is always best to replace a rainforest with a rainforest and not replace a rainforest with monoculture. Yes, if you wipe out all of your microbiome with antibiotics it might make sense to take probiotics for a period of time because to have something is better than to have nothing. But for one's day-to-day needs, it is important to live a lifestyle that naturally replenishes the microbiome by living in community and by eating healthy rather than to rely on monoculture to keep you healthy.

The Five Protocols I recommend are based on killing specific sets of infectious organisms. Some of these protocols have overlapping tools, which means you can get double the benefits if you use them. The goal of each protocol is not to permanently kill off all of the stated organisms in your system because that is impossible. It is also not possible to get rid of every last individual of any of these organisms from your body. These are smart infectious organisms in their own way and they have strategies perfected over billions of years as to how to chronically infect, not all of which we can counter with these Protocols alone. Instead, the Protocols are meant to keep the populations of these pathogens at low levels so that they are effectively asymptomatic and also not large enough in quantity as to damage tissues to any significant degree.

The "ad hoc" use of these protocols is when you have had a known exposure and so you then employ a protocol to address that exposure at that immediate moment in time rather than waiting for it to come up in the calendar. I strongly recommend you make use of these protocols ad hoc in this way. The longer you let an infection fester, the harder it is to clear it. The faster you respond, the better your results.

Think of the calendar as trying to reduce chronic infections over time whereas the ad hoc use of these Protocols are strategies to keep you from getting any new infections that might threaten to become chronic. Ad hoc is therefore used to deal with your immediate threats and the calendar is meant to over time reduce your overall load of latent infections you are likely not even aware that you have.

This is very important: when using the protocols "ad hoc," follow the number of days recommended within the protocol. When applying a protocol for the stated month on the calendar, follow the protocol for 30 days and ignore the number of days stated in this chapter.

A "Herxheimer Reaction" is a state of fatigue, achiness, irritability, and/or foggy headedness that results when so many white blood cells stream through the lymphatic system to clear the debris of dead pathogens and their toxins that the lymphatic fluid stagnates. It is likely that at times, when applying these strategies, you might find yourself experiencing a Herxheimer Reaction. The number one best cure for this is to drink more plain water (not even lemon or lime added), as the lymphatic fluid prefers to be flush with water to operate efficiently.

The human body has a necessary enzyme for detoxing pathogen toxins that is called MTHFR enzyme that helps to make something called glutathione. Many people have a single broken gene for making MTHFR enzyme and some people have both genes broken and do not make this enzyme. If you do not know your status of your genes around this enzyme and find that a Herxheimer reaction is lasting more than 3 days, then it is a good idea for you to take supplemental glutathione to help you detox the pathogen toxins that might be released into your system by organisms popping and dying. If you are someone who has suffered chronic fatigue and/or has been very frequently sick since you were a child, I highly recommend that you assume you have two broken MTHFR enzymes and that the first four days of every protocol you initiate, that you take supplemental glutathione so that you can clear pathogen toxins and not feel fatigued or depleted each time you follow these Protocols.

Anti-Fungal Protocol and Anaerobic Protocol

Fungal pathogens and anaerobic bacteria/fungi are considered "Damp Pathogens" in Chinese medicine, which means they live in Damp environments and promote the build-up of energetic Dampness in the body. Over my career, I have come to find that Damp environments are the same thing as "low-oxygen" environments and that by increasing the level of oxygen in your system, you rob these organisms of the environment in which they need to live, resulting in their die off.

Nettle Tea (Stinging Nettle Tea)

Recommended Dose:
3 cups a day for two weeks

What This Is:
The Stinging Nettle plant is found worldwide. It has hairs filled with highly irritating compounds in its natural state. However, in its herbal form, the compounds within this herb are highly oxygenating. It also has natural anti-histamine properties.

Why We Use Nettle Tea:
Damp energy is a low oxygen state and when you introduce stinging nettle to the body, it dramatically increases oxygen in the body, clearing out this Dampness. Pathogens that require Dampness to survive die off in abundance.

- Or -

Pomegranate Extract

Recommended Dose:
250mg twice daily for two weeks

What This Is:
Pomegranate extract is a concentrated powder form of mainly the skin of the pomegranate fruit. Pomegranate fruit is high in anti-oxidants and has many bio-active properties.

Why We Use Pomegranate Extract:
Pomegranate boosts immune function while clearing free radicals.

- Or -

Hyperbaric Oxygen Chamber

Recommended Use:
Every 3 days for 3 instances

What This Is:
Hyperbaric oxygen is a service often available in cities where one is exposed to very high oxygen for a period of time – often 30 minutes to multiple hours.

Why We Use Hyperbaric Oxygen:
Exposure to high oxygen environments will clear Dampness from the body and will therefore kill off Damp Pathogens. Beware of upselling by the purveyors of these services as often additional remedies such as ozone injections and other therapeutics are provided at these same service centers. I recommend sticking to the oxygen chambers for now.

- Or -

Caprylic Acid

Recommended Dose:
600mg or more twice a day for 2 weeks

What This Is:
Caprylic acid, also known as octanoic acid, is a natural medium-chain fatty acid found in many natural oils and animal milks. While it has anti-inflammatory benefits, our main focus is in its anti-microbial and specifically yeast killing properties.

Why We Use Caprylic Acid:
This is a very powerful tool for killing off yeasts very specifically, and yeasts are fast growing forms of Damp Pathogens that we are all exposed to regularly even if we do not eat bread, as they are often ambient in the air or passed person to person readily.

- Or -

Oregano Oil (Oil Of Oregano)

Recommended Daily Dose:
10 tincture drops in water twice a day for 2 weeks (or as recommended by other medical practitioners)

What This Is:
Oil of oregano is a liquid extract from wild oregano. I do **not** recommend this for people with sensitive skin as it can cause rashes in people who suffer from persistent high histamine levels. I recommend starting with only 3 drops to see if you tolerate it before increasing to 10.

Why We Use Oregano Oil:
This oil has very specific anti-fungal properties and is often used therapeutically to address overgrowth of yeast, including Candida.

- Or -

Apple Cider Vinegar

Recommended Dose:
1 tablespoon mixed with water before each meal for 14 days

What This Is:
Apple cider vinegar is fermented apple cider, which is full of acetic acid.

Why We Use Apple Cider Vinegar:
Even though the process to make apple cider vinegar involves yeast and bacteria, it is thought that this form of vinegar, due to the acetic acid, has unusually strong anti-fungal properties.

Anti-Bacterial Protocol

Bacterial pathogens tend not to infect cells and tend to produce robust colonies on the body's exterior surfaces and internal tubing. If one develops a mouth, tongue, lip, or cheek ulcer, do not assume it is Herpes Simplex, instead saturate a cotton ball or "q-tip" with 3% hydrogen peroxide and hold it against the ulcer for 60 seconds, as it is likely this is actually a bacterial colony attempting to colonize the skin or mucus membranes.

Goldenseal Root Herb

Recommended Dose:
700mg to 1g capsules twice a day for 2 weeks.

What This Is:
Goldenseal, Hydrastis Canadensis, is a dried herbal root from the buttercup family, which is high in berberine.

[s](Age) Age Backwards

Why We Use Goldenseal Root:
Berberine is thought to be a potent anti-microbial agent which can be used to kill bacteria and fungi, though I tend to recommend it for bacterial pathogens primarily. Please note that there are known drug/herb interactions with this herb, so I recommend reviewing medicines with which it interacts should you be on any medications.

- Or -

Colloidal Silver

Recommended Dose:
1 teaspoon 4 times a day for 4 days (do not take colloidal silver for more than 14 days in a row)

What This Is:
This fluid solution contains very small silver particles suspended in water. While Western medicine does not feel there is any therapeutic benefit from this modality and claims it is unsafe, practitioners of alternative self-care have used this tool for decades and swear by its effectiveness against bacterial pathogens in particular.

Why We Use Colloidal Silver:
Silver is thought to have anti-microbial properties. Colloidal silver can interfere with the absorption of some medications and so make sure any medicine you are taking does not have any known interaction effects with it. Too much silver can cause permanent discoloration of the skin, but if used according to the directions on its bottle (no longer than 14 days in a row – and here I recommend only 4 days in our protocol), this should not be an issue.

- Or -

Elderberry Syrup

Recommended Dose:
Follow the bottle's instructions for daily dosage up to 2 weeks.

What This Is:
This syrup is made from the berries of the Sambucus tree and has been used for hundreds of years across the world to boost the immune system as a classical herbal tool for self-care. It is very high in vitamin C.

Why We Use Elderberry:
Elderberry helps boost the immune system and is fabulous for boosting immunity in real-time when there are acute exposures (whereas Echinacea and astragalus need weeks to build up their respective immune benefits, by way of comparison). It is also used in the Anti-Viral Protocol, as it is known to reduce the length and severity of viral infections such as colds and flues as well.

Anti-Viral Protocol

Viruses are hard to clear because they infect internal to cells. It is much harder to disrupt processes occurring behind cell walls, to the benefit of viruses that have successfully penetrated our cellular barrier tissue. Echinacea is a protective against infection, but not a method of clearing active infections. Except for elderberry, the suggestions below are primarily Chinese herbs, used for hundreds of years to eradicate viruses.

Elderberry Syrup

See the recommendations above in the Anti-Bacterial Protocol

- Or -

[8](Age) Age Backwards

Minced Ginger Tea

Recommended Dose:
Two cups a day for 14 days. Mince the ginger root into small pieces or a few thin cross sections and put in hot water. Let steep 5 minutes or more.

What This Is:
Ginger root is a classic Chinese medical herb used for a wide variety of health issues, including “releasing the exterior” which is our protocol for fending off acute viral infections.

Why We Use Ginger:
Ginger warms and releases the exterior, which can induce sweating, which is a key facet of the Chinese medical strategy for clearing viral infections.

- Or -

Spring Onion Tea

Recommended Dose:
One cup of tea up to three times a day (once if not fending off an infection but two or three times depending on your level of viral exposure or if you are at the beginning of acute infection symptoms – ie. “feeling off”).

What This Is:
Spring onions are the long thin mostly green onions easily found in supermarkets. Cut up the entire length of the onion and use all of it. Wash thoroughly to clear any pesticides before steeping in hot water to remove any pesticides.

Why We Use Spring Onion:
Spring onion tea will induce sweating which is a key strategy in

Chinese medicine in fending off viral infections. We especially prefer this strategy when one is acutely being attacked in the early stages of an infection or when there has been an exposure to pathogens but no symptoms yet.

- Or -

Astragalus Root Tincture

Recommended Dose:
Follow the instructions on the bottle for 30 days

What This Is:
This is a tincture made up of Astragalus root, a classic Chinese herb. Astragalus is an "adaptogen," which means it is generally good for the body in maintaining homeostasis.

Why We Use Astragalus:
In Chinese medicine, we have an energy called "Wei Qi" that makes up the immune system. Astragalus uniquely builds up Wei Qi and so it is very specifically great at fending off viral infections (and other infections). Building up Wei Qi takes time and so one needs to be on astragalus for an extended period of time to maximize its immune strengthening benefits, which is why our protocol requires 30 days of use.

- Or -

Garlic Capsules

Recommended Dose:
3000 or more milligrams a day up to 3 times a day for up to 30 days

What This Is:
These are dried tablets or capsules of garlic, full of allicin, a sulfur-rich compound.

Why We Use Garlic:
Garlic is a Chinese medical herb with many properties, but the one we care about here is its ability to fend off infections. It is known that ajoene and allin, sulfur containing compounds, disrupt the cellular processes of many infectious organisms.

Anti-Parastic Protocol

Parasites are complex organisms that can be difficult to eradicate. They often have different life stages and most interventions do not tend to address each of these equally, which is why herbs do not sustainably kill most parasites.

Over The Counter Pinworm Medicines

Recommended Dose:
Utilize over-the-counter pinworm medicines according to their instructions. Often, one dose is taken and three weeks later a second dose is required to clear whatever has hatched from eggs in the interim.

What This Is:
Pinworm medicines are anthelmintic (anti-parasite) medicines, often containing pyrantel pamoate as the active therapeutic ingredient.

Why We Use Pinworm Remedies:
Pinworm infects more than 11% of the human population at any given moment in time, as one of the most successful infectious multi-cellular organisms on the planet. Not only will this medicine kill pinworms, I have found it often kills off Demodex mites, which usually are

symbiotic with us but can turn infectious and lead to massive bone loss due to mineral malabsorption. These organisms are particularly problematic in causing osteopenia and osteoporosis. Furthermore, these medicines tend to be very mild on the system and very well tolerated.

- Or -

Artemesia Mugwort Tincture

Recommended Dose:
Follow directions on the bottle for 30 days (there are other Chinese medical applications that can be recommended to you by a Chinese herbalist)

What This is:
Artemesia Mugwort is one of the most important herbs in Chinese medicine, as it is often burnt on or around the body via a popular technique called Moxibustion. In our protocol, we are utilizing a different property of this herb – which its strong ability to clear gu (multi-cellular parasites) from the body.

Why We Use Artemesia Mugwort:
This herb has been used for hundreds, if not thousands of years as an anthelmintic.

- Or -

Black Walnut With Wormwood Tincture

Recommended Dose:
Follow the direction on the bottle for 30 days

What This Is:
Black Walnut is the unripe hull of Juglans nigra tree but also can include its leaves and bark which have similar therapeutic properties. The napthoquinones in black walnut are thought to inhibit necessary enzymes for parasite survival. Other molecules in this herb such as tannins can help expel parasites.

Wormwood, known as Artemesia Absinthium, contains thujone and other compounds thought to be antiparasitic by way of weakening the cell walls of parasites, creating vulnerabilities to the human immune system.

Why We Use Black Walnut and Wormwood:
These herbs utilize different, complimentary techniques in weakening and killing off a wide range of parasites.

Are These Protocol Enough?

My goal is not to cure you of every ailment with this book because this is not a book of cures and you are a unique person who needs a professional health care practitioner following your situation to make the best calls on what you need. A professional has books of knowledge stored in their intellect with many strategies and interventions for many unique applications. What I am offering you, however, is a highly reductive path that is meant to simplify self-care strategies that will meet a large population's regular needs in broad strokes. I strongly encourage you to take what I have offered here as a path on which you can run that might carry you to people who take a deep health history intake and offer more direct interventions for specific factors in your life – especially once you start to see the benefits of employing these strategies and you start to turn back the clock on aging. If you find you there are protocols that are not quite hitting your needs for problems I have outlined in this book, I strongly encourage you to then find a trained professional to find out how to unlock those factors for your unique body. For instance, if I have indicated that parasites are a common factor in a particular issue and you don't seem to be making progress with the above Anti-Parasitic protocols, go to a doctor, naturopath, osteopath, Chinese medical herbalist, homeopath, or so many other possible sharp minds with good hearts that want to see you make progress and feel more youthful and less symptomatic.

Who I Was

It is 1992. I am at Harvey Mudd College sitting outdoors, my back against a classroom building, warming like a lizard in the sun. I am two years into what I would later self-diagnose as chronic Lyme Disease, a syndrome very few people discussed in the late 90s and the "chronic" part still to this day disputed by insurance companies that do not want to pay for its remediation. I have spent the last two years in an angstful depression. I am taking a light semester of classes on purpose, as a way to recover from two grueling years at Swarthmore College where I had to fight my body every day to get my challenging school work completed. I wanted my time in California to include self-reflection. This is the moment. I decide to revisit my life story.

I am sitting stunned. I can't remember my past. I can't remember high school. I can't remember my childhood. It is akin to amnesia except that I haven't forgotten myself and I know I have a past, I just can't find it in my memory banks. It is sad and terrifying. I know I had what most people would consider a very good childhood, close friends, travel and adventures, and strangely enough my high school years were bearable, even enjoyable. But I can't remember a thing. Not a single moment.

I force myself to remember, willing total recall. But it is like quick sand. I am sinking. My mind is empty. There is nothing there. I am stranded on a memory island where only the last two years remain cogent.

And yet, I am lucky. Over the ensuing years, it does all come back.

1998 was the year I decided to become a practitioner of Chinese medicine. Eastern, not Western medicine guided me out of seven years of chronic fatigue. I was not yet 100% at that moment of this decision, but there was light at the end of the tunnel. I temporarily considered becoming a naturopathic doctor, having experienced naturopathy as an alternative form of Western medicine and benefited from it. As I said, I was pre-med in college but by the end of college decided to write poetry instead. Shocking no one, poetry didn't pay my bills, so I stuck my thumb out on the side of the road as a "will-write -for-money" copywriter. This was 1994 when Netscape suddenly showed every business on the planet that if they did not join the "World Wide Web" with a website, they would be left behind in tatters. Absolute panic ensued. Copywriting soon led me to writing HTML to meet this sudden WWW obsession – HTML being the programming language for the internet. Soon, I was a programmer making mind blowing sums of money (to me) writing the first website and intranets for such notable Fortune 500 companies such as Merrill Lynch, Ikon, Jannsen Pharmaceuticals, and more as a contract worker working as a programmer-for-hire through a Temp agency. When I signed up to program not only did I not know how much website programmers made per hour, neither did the Temp agency. I proposed $55 per hour and to my great surprise, they hired me and kept hiring me. I suddenly felt like the richest poet of all time.

I became a programmer of languages other than HTML and wrote Visual Basic programs, Javascript, Coldfusion, Java, and more. I sold the intellectual rights of one program I had created for my own recently created business and it paid for my next two years working out of my side room in a rented house in Seattle as my soon-to-be wife, Jen, finished her first Masters Degree. Those two years were a roller coaster. They were in what is now known as the Dot Com Boom – or more appropriately the Dot Com Bubble. As a member of several startups, there were moments of extreme excitement where one day I thought I was going to be a millionaire and the next day realized I was still making maybe $15,000 a year (no longer my original $55/hr wage) plus a percentage of one company or another worth zero.

By the end of those years, I was offered an opportunity from a colleague to move to the San Francisco area to make six figures at a large tech company, keep on going nowhere with startups, or pivot massively out of this absolutely insanity. I chose the massive pivot. During those two years, I slowly realized that I still really cared tremendously about healthcare, but was no longer attracted to Western medicine. Ergo, I looked at naturopathy, what I consider an alternative form of Western medicine. And the more I looked at naturopathy, the more I realized I was actually far more interested in Chinese medicine, what would only be a fraction of a Naturopath's education.

When I decided to become an acupuncturist, I lost all of my high school friends. You could say that it was just a moment of expiration, a facet of dissolving nature of time. However, the timing appeared to me to be very specific. Back in 1998, acupuncture was nowhere near mainstream. It was a strange choice. It made me look strange to my mainstream friends, which brings me even deeper into my past.

I grew up a white, middle class, suburbinite in a city that is very salt of the Earth, Rochester, NY. My childhood was 1970s and 1980s mainstream suburban. My family ate red meat and highly processed American food. We rarely traveled internationally – mainly to Florida, Cape Cod, and nearby Toronto. My school friends wrote for the yearbook and school newspaper and cared about their grades. They worked hard to get into Ivy League schools. When I wasn't doing homework, I was playing catch, shooting hoops, arguing over touch football, or working my way up the local rankings in tennis. I was a little league All Star every year that I played. I lost only one tennis match in my four years of High School tennis and ranked 3rd in the region for my age. I was exactly what you would expect I would be. Square. Meat and potatoes.

My dad is a physician who worked hard in his field to build an amazing reputation. I had every expectation of following his path into a field that focused on helping people overcome their health challenges and thrive. I really enjoyed my science classes and worked Summers in a DNA lab and at my dad's medical office while acing Summer Organic Chemistry classes at the University of Rochester.

When I chose to become an acupuncturist, my parents wondered why I didn't become an acupuncturist and also a physician. I get it. Why go so far off field when you have a talent for natural sciences and Western medicine is "in the family?" I guess my high school friends must have felt the same way. One by one, they disappeared. We had once been thick as thieves and now I felt abandoned but also undeterred. There was something pulling me towards Chinese medicine: my purpose. On the one hand, my heart felt broken. On the other, my heart found its meaning.

It is the day I choose to become an acupuncturist. I am driving home from the Open House of what will become decades later the National College of Natural Medicine in Portland, Oregon. I randomly bump into a former Swarthmore College friend who is in his second year at this school. He is in the middle of his finals and he is stressed, burnt out, and distraught. He strongly discourages me from attending. The moment seems fated. I am driving home ruminating on the different segments of the National College's program and again and again I find myself gravitating towards the Chinese medicine lecture. I started receiving acupuncture as a patient while living in Media, Pennsylvania four years prior and after the very first session I felt energy movement in my abdomen that made absolutely no sense at all from an anatomical perspective. It was going round and round in circles clockwise in my abdomen at tremendous speed and it was not subtle. I realize, if the only part of naturopathy that interests me is Chinese medicine, why not go to a school that focuses only on this? As soon as I think this, I know this is my path.

But that's not the weird part. The weird part is the thousands of tiny dots that suddenly fill my visual field. I have never seen or noticed them before in my life – ever. But they suddenly appear everywhere and are impossible to ignore. It is not instantaneous at the moment of this decision, but they make their way into my consciousness over the ensuing hours and days.

I can't unsee them. Actually, I find myself quite alarmed. It is as if my visual field has behind it the pixelated noise of a color television. I am wondering if I am suddenly losing my vision, but my vision remains unchanged as the days and weeks and months progress. It takes me years to stop focusing on these colorful pixels in my visual field, though they never go away. It is my first day of seeing energy. It starts the day I decide my fate. Through my Chinese medicine education it remains a mystery and a reminder – there is more out there than I understand.

Who I Am

It is 2002, in May. It is snowing in Boston. I am speaking at my New England School of Acupuncture graduation. I am nervous, but I was also a speaker at my high school graduation, so I am using an old trick and taking deep breaths to activate my parasympathetic system. I am sweating as the moment approaches. I do not yet realize that my life will be full of public speaking, as a facet of doing something different than the norm and therefore having something interesting to say that people have a hunger to hear. My speech is a humorous review of the long road to a three year graduate degree in classical medicine. I talk about mixing herbs together like a pure scientist and its unexpected bowel side effects. I talk about needling oranges as a beginning beginner and my appreciation to the humans who "chose" (chose may be too strong of a word, perhaps were bribed) to immediately be next in line from an actual orange on one's needling journey – and the many family and friend guinea pigs that followed. My speech is over. I feel relief. This is not just relief of finishing a public talk I had anxiously anticipated, but the relief of having finished a leg of a long journey that finally brought me to a vista from which I could see how worth it was the toil and struggle. As I see it, it was very worth the toil and struggle – which in no way minimizes how toiling was the toil and how struggling was the struggle.

In 1999, I finally healed myself of 7 years of chronic fatigue while in acupuncture school. In college, as you know, I had decided I would have to be the one who solved my issue and in the end, with some contributions here and there from others. My goal was achieved years later and, in true fashion, I did most of the intellectual and physical labor myself. Working on the Kidney meridian and especially the Earth Qi points on this meridian and also on the Spleen and Stomach meridians. This finally solved what lingered, ending a very long, painful episode in my life. By 2002, I had more energy than the average adult and I have had more energy than the above average adult for the ensuing two and a half decades, decades I have worked as a professional in the field of Chinese medicine day in/day out with gusto.

In 2002, I graduated from the New England School of Acupuncture as a Chinese medical herbalist and Japanese style acupuncturist. Over the ensuing years, my back of the envelope estimate is that I have facilitated more than 40,000 patient visits – working on an average of 10 patients a day and an average of 4.5 working days a week. The beginning years were a quiet, lonely struggle but once I started treating people with medical Qi Gong, my practice built itself by reputation and it has remained highly caffeinated to this day – for which I feel tremendously blessed and highly appreciative.

Since graduation, I have written over 20 books, mostly in my field and a majority of these books expounding on classical Chinese energy medicine intermixed with my own obsessive exploration bridging the gap between classical theory and modern ideas of anatomy and physiology.

In 2010, I produced a product line based on classical Chinese energy medicine called Qi Infusions which I have sold in regional health food stores and in my own online seasonal "pop-up" store. It has over 20 products ranging a very wide gamut of physical, emotional, and even spiritual health complaints.

In 2013, I began teaching my unique method of energy medicine, Eminus Mirus (which means "astonishing at a distance"), to health practitioners and lay people. I have taught 100s of people all four levels of my method, which expands from a simple, free method at Level 1 to thousands upon thousands of pages of complex, exciting theory with multiple, profound diagnostic methods unique to this medical art.

In 2021, I started Energy Medicine Urgent Care, based on Western medicine urgent care centers (found in the United States) for same day emergency care, but utilizing my classical energy medicine as the treatment vehicle. I will note, this service is not for Western medical emergencies such as strokes, heart attacks, gushing wounds, etc, but for everyday "emergencies" where same day care is a much better idea than waiting for one's next healthcare appointment days, weeks, or months down the road.

I believe it is fair to say that I have top notch professional level experience within my field – an expert in my domain, a master of medical Qi Gong, and, uniquely, an innovator in a medicine that is perhaps 6000 years old. I will also add that I have done this quietly, not seeking fame or fortune. I am just a guy putting his head down and pushing forward every day – doing the hard grind of helping as many people as possible with the time I have on planet. I am a healer. That is my purpose.

Despite being prolific, this is my first book that I have written with mass market aspirations. I have written it because I have reached a point in my career with enough perspective on enough people to add some new ideas to the conversation that might just reduce suffering for you and many others. Sometimes the best way to heal as many people as possible is not with needles or herbs, but ink on paper. If just one idea in here helps you, my job is complete. But if more than one idea helps you or inspires you, perhaps you should share this book written by a caring healer (with a fifteen year old Prius) with a best friend or family member, or maybe your book club. Yes, definitely your book club. Possibly we recall Oprah and she shares it with her book club.

I know, I'm being glib. But if you read the above, you can see I worked hard for at least one free shameless plug. If your version of this book, at the end of the day, is dog-eared, annotated, and sitting on your neighbor's bedside table, then I have achieved my goal, perhaps with a new view from a new vista, another leg of a long journey completed. Goal achieved. Hallelujah and also amen!

Dying

I am 12 years old at Ramah Island, a little island we canoed to for our cabin's overnight adventure. My belly is full of blueberries which I have picked all across the island, naturally growing on the algae and moss covered boulders covering the petite island landscape from which giant pine trees abound.

We are swimming in the chilly Canadian waters, laughing our asses off. It is the early 1980s. For a white, middle class, suburbanite at Summer camp, life seems sublime. There is an overhanging pine tree above the water. I decide I should climb up so that I can jump into the water. I am sopping wet and in no way does this cross my mind. The pine tree is a natural ladder where I can climb a couple of feet up limb to limb. I go higher and higher. Water is dripping down the sides of my shirt as I extend my arms up to the next limb. My hands are damp. I am fifteen feet above a very large boulder. My hands suddenly slip at the same time my feet glide free. For a millisecond, I am falling. The tree is a natural ladder and my athletic reflexes kick in. My body has a natural desire to live. Evolution must have spun this story before, as it works without consciousness. I am airborne – totally free, bound only by gravity and, as a consequence, a meeting with a vast block of sharp quartzite seemingly intended below. But somehow like a miracle I grab the next branch down and hold on for dear life. The moist hands hold – perhaps the power of wet fingerpad wrinkles, sparing me from hitting the boulder and crashing into the water with a broken body. My heart beats out of my body. I know what I just escaped. But I tell no one. I feel a tremendous sense of embarrassment, shame, and humiliation – even though the episode apparently had not one single witness. I climb down the tree safely and perhaps this is the first etch or maybe a second or third in a fear of heights that one day leaves me shaking on a bridge in Cincinnati decades later.

My body is prepared to fight like heck for life, that's for sure. It has a programmed intelligence to seek safety and fear harm. But my mind sees death as a redistribution of energy, a change of state, permanent for this body but impermanent for the energy, which perhaps has many forms it would like to take before the full yarn has unraveled.

I am born. I have no recollection of being afraid in any existence prior to my being me. I therefore see no reason being afraid of my existence when I am me no more.

Perhaps dying is over-rated. We tend to spend a plethora of life energy on the subject – not just the existence and shape of a hereafter but on the many nasty shapes dying can take. There is no doubt that it takes many forms, most of which seem unpleasant. But then again, dying is a single act and life is full of hopefully decades of far more interesting acts and episodes. It therefore seems a shame we spend so much life force on the topic of dying.

Then again, there are reasons why we cannot ignore dying. First, as noted in my anecdote, the body believes it should not die. And it reminds us at certain common enough moments – such as being dangerously cut off by another driver, with a dry mouth when public speaking, at moments of vulnerability of the heart when professing one's love for the first time, and more. Our bodies can be raging hormone machines that communicate with blood pressure, sweat, and lightheadedness a biological refrain: "I want to live!"

We also cannot escape thinking about dying because people die. We hear their stories regularly. We live in a global community of worldwide celebrity and people we do not personally know die all the time – let alone the people we do know and personally mourn. Death is part of the news cycle. News is narrative and humans are narrative creatures who have used stories since the dawn of time to communicate all kinds of important factoids about life and living and also therefore death and dying. We gobble up all of this news and the deaths of people far and wide swim in our swells of consciousness. Rarely are these stories uplifting and life affirming.

There is yet another reason we think so much of dying and in fact, a reason that increases as we age. You might think I am talking about our aging bodies, which obviously do communicate the natural changes the body endures as we cross different genetic epochs. But I am not. I am talking about anaerobic pathogens that grow increasingly inside us. These are organisms that live in scar tissue that, through the toxins they produce, increase within us thoughts about our own mortality. They increase anxiety and dread. The older we get, the more these organisms and their toxins build up and it becomes harder and harder to ignore the bell that rings only once in our lives.

While it is clear that we cannot stop our natural, native human biology that reminds us from time to time with a racing heart that we should value our lives, there are actually things we can do to stop dwelling on death and dying and focus on the more immediately important facets of living, dreaming, and achieving.

First, read the news, don't watch it. Video news is designed to invoke narratives with more dimension, utilizing fear-inducing, thunderous music and the evocative nature of hosts and their guests via tone, emotion, and powerful language with the goal of grabbing and squeezing our narrative-loving hearts. Written news doesn't do any of this. It just gives us details without the music and without kabuki theater. Read the news. I cannot tell you how powerful an intervention this is in reducing anxiety in the modern era. Powerful and simple.

Second, kill anaerobic pathogens from your body. It is a good idea to do this every 6 months after you turn fifty (or earlier, ad hoc, if you are noticing that fear of dying is more present in your thoughts). "Anaerobic" means these are organisms that live in low or no oxygen environments. You can think of these organisms as if they are the bottom feeders of the eco-system. They are the necessary tools for tearing apart dead cells and recycling the energy stored within these cells back into a living biological biome. We need anaerobes on this planet as they play an important, fundamental ecological role. But what we don't need are organisms trying to recycle us while we are still alive. Anaerobes die off in high oxygen environments. Oxygen is highly reactive and we cannot live in too high of an oxygen environment as this encourages free radical formation which is bad for health. But we can use oxygen as a tool periodically, which is why I suggest every 6 months generating a very high oxygen environment in your body to obliterate organisms in your ecosystem that promote more scar tissue formation and more tissue degredation.

There are two ways to do this that I utilize in my work with patients. I'm sure there are other strategies out there that you might discover and perhaps enjoy even more.

1. The expensive method: hyperbaric oxygen chambers. These expose you to high oxygen levels for an hour or so. Often, these are run by people who are happy enough to encourage you to buy packages and keep returning every week or so, which I do not recommend. Once or once a week up to three weeks every 6 months, like a dental cleaning is ideal
2. The cheap way (my personal preference): nettle tea, as in tea made from "stinging nettles." You can find tea made from nettles in the United States in every health food store and almost every grocery store with a large tea section. Drink 2 cups a day for three weeks. This creates a high oxygen environment internally and at very little expense

Death is a bookend of life and there is no escaping that. But there is also no need to dwell on it to a degree that feels unbalanced or anxiety provoking. It is important to not fear death and dying and allow it to occupy more of your consciousness during this unique opportunity to both "be" and "become," that you should wholeheartedly embrace.

Instead, one can think of dying as an inevitable part of a journey where you reach a point where you free your energy, releasing it back into the cosmos that made you. One thing that is true about energy is that it likes to move and wants to move. It has a propensity to move and its nature is movement. Therefore, what a blessing that it gives us decades accumulated in our physical form. At some point, however, you will need to release this energy and allow it to be free and flow, to return to the entropy that is its nature.

Our culture says death and dying is bad and for sure it is sad for us that we as individuals must one day go. But for our energy, it is a freedom we will one day grant it. And while one should not run hastily into the void, when the time comes, you will be giving a gift to the energy that comprises you when you free it. From my perspective, this makes the end not an entirely terrible thing, since this energy has served you in so many ways and has given you so many blessings as a consequence of "being." It is your final act of giving. And while this giving has been pre-programmed into the experience, you can embrace this as a conscious and meaningful act when the time eventually arises. Or not. That is entirely up to you.

The Meaning Of Life

It's 1990. I have my eyes on a cute freshman at Swarthmore College who happens to live on my hall. She has been playing soccer all Autumn and finally her season is over and there is a chance to connect. We are at a "Go Go Go" improv group performance together with other hallmates. The performance is ending and I'm hungry. I ask everyone within earshot if they want to join me at Tarbles, the college cafe, for a snack. One by one, I'm turned down until we get to cutie. Cutie says "yes." A shot of adrenaline spikes through me.

It is dark out on a cold late October night in Pennsylvania. As we walk towards Tarbles, both she and I spot a giant pile of leaves in the middle of the grounds. It happens spontaneously. We both shout: "leaves!" at the same time. We both run towards the giant pile and dive in. It is at least three feet tall and ten feet wide, enveloping us in its embrace.

The leaves are warm under the frosted top layers. Who knows what else is under this canopy with us wriggling around and who cares? We toss leaves at each other and laugh. We talk and talk. An hour later, Tarbles is closed and we are still talking. We decide to go back to our dorm and make tea because now we are shivering. Later, I learn that my interest in Cinnamon Vienna tea distinguished me as a gentleman.

It is 1999, nine years later. We are in an adorable Meeting House in Damariscotta, Maine yards from the beautiful, craggily coast. It is raining outside, but who cares? Cutie and I are under the "chuppa," a traditional shawl held up by my cousins. I am stomping down, breaking a glass, another traditional act in a Jewish wedding. Cutie glows. She is the most beautiful person on the planet.

My heart is full of light. This is living.

Most of life is not like this. This is peak. Most of life is not peak, which I guess is what makes peak "peak." Some moments stand out like gold in a prospector's pan but honestly most moments are just the rest of the crud in that pan. Most of life is walking the dog and cleaning her grimy water bowl. Most of life is a moment of indigestion that flits into consciousness. Most of life is putting sunglasses on because it's suddenly blinding.

Most of life is wading through empty space from one act of work to the next responsible "act of daily living." We like to think that life is full of exclamations but in reality much of life is the empty space between letters. There is a banality to existence – and this is if you are lucky. If you are unlucky, life is a trudge through muddier, more dangerous waters in more dangerous and desolute places. Billions of people on this planet lack adequate access to water. Some people walk miles to fill jugs of water from the closest watering hole. Most of their days are walking under the weight of what keeps them alive.

So why do we do it? Why do we put up with ruts that deepen as we age? What is the true meaning of life?

My answer would be a spiritual answer – something about fate and destiny – which speaks to a higher power and higher purpose. To another person, those might just be mumbo-jumbo words that carry no magnetic force. This book is not about trying to convince anyone to carry my beliefs like a jug of water five miles down the road. Instead, I offer practical ideas you can simply test and see if they work. If you like the real life impacts of my suggestions and my thinking behind why I suggest them, you can keep repeating the procedures. If you don't, no harm done.

To the most part I won't get into the fire that propels me forward every day, through weeks and months that sometimes share little nuance. Which is to say, though this book is based on the work of a medical intuitive, unlike other books by medical intuitives, you do not have to have any spiritual framework at all to join me on this jouney, let alone one in alignment with my own, to find utility on these pages.

Often, when I read similar books, I find myself immediately at odds with the writer because I don't agree with the author's foundational beliefs that meander into spirits and souls, religious doctrine of a certain faith, and whatnot. I am living my truths and they seem to be working well for me – different truths than these other authors. Which says to me, perhaps this is not the right venue to talk about spiritual things because my only goal is provide you practical utility. I don't want my truths and your truths to feel incompatible and for this to be a reason to stop before we start.

What is living? I leave that up to you. Why fight to keep on living? I leave that up to you. What is the meaning behind the veil? I leave that up to you. If some of my beliefs creep in here by accident, please forgive me and also understand that your beliefs and mine do not have to match and yet I might still say something useful worth consideration. I honor your journey and how you have come to make sense of it. My only goal is to provide some valuable practices that might keep your journey ongoing and with the least possible suffering.

Thriving & "More Thrive-y"

It is 2017. We are meeting up with my wife's brother and fiance in Cincinnati. We are staying in Kentucky, just across the river. In order to cross this river, we walk over a bridge. The bridge is not super tall but there is no actual bottom of the bridge. It is made of slatted metal leaving large gaping holes to stare straight through into the river below. I have a terrible bridge phobia that turned full on the very day I likely got Lyme disease, 27 years earlier. How they correlate, I have my suspicions but am not entirely certain. But that doesn't matter at this moment, because nothing matters because I am literally terrified. My children, brother-in-law and his fiance are ahead of me walking at a normal steady pace. My wife is walking with me as I slow down more and more, decelerating from normal pace to half pace and now to a crawl – from the sheer terror that is building cement inside of my legs. My heart is racing and I am light headed. I have passed the point of no return. It is just as much a terror to go backwards as it is to go forwards, as it requires crossing the same distance of this floating horror. My wife holds my hand and speaks encouraging words. I force myself to keep moving. It is agony, but eventually we make it to the other side. I am a sweaty wreck, but I have crossed the rubicon and survived.

We make it to the museum. It is a museum on the history of slavery in the United States and the resilience of African Americans. For more than an astonishing 250 years people were "owned," beaten, terrorized, and dehumanized up and down the Americas. Yet they found a way to persevere...not for hours or days, not for years or decades, but for centuries. Slaves created a dancing form of martial arts in Brazil. They created songs that hid messages to communicate what otherwise could not be said. They created heroes, freed slaves who put their lives in peril to return to unshackle others. And then they found freedom, full citizenship, and resplendent democratic power. It is truly a testament to the human spirit.

On the way back to Rochester from Cincinnati, I am driving home. The bridge episode has raised my baseline levels of fight or flight hormones way higher than normal. I don't often have panic attacks driving on highways outside of bridges but I find myself in the driver's seat spiking another panic attack. My kids are unaware, but my wife knows because suddenly I am driving like an idiot accelarating then hitting the breaks in a jerky, speed up/slow down staccato, a normal pattern when I am crossing a bridge. I find myself highly afraid to drive in the 2nd and 3rd lanes. I find myself terrified to pass trucks. This episode resonates in my heart like a loss of pride and dignity, a bell that keeps ringing every time I drive for a very very long time thereafter. But here's the thing: I love to drive. It is a meditative space for me. I won't be giving up driving. When we are back in Rochester, I get in the car and I force myself to drive in the 2nd and 3rd lanes. I force myself to pass trucks. I go out again and again. It doesn't take hours or days or even weeks, it takes months and years but I break through some secret threshold in my heart and release the fear. I can drive again freely at any speed in any lane but even now I still hear that bell – it still rings, but I cope.

Life is not always fun but it also happens to be the only life we have at this moment (possibilities of reincarnation aside). In my faith, this is your one and done and so it is meant to be enjoyed as much as one can. And yet, life is not always a joy ride. Indignities abound. I cannot tell you how many times my pant's fly has been down while out in public all day long, how many times I have spent hours talking face-to-face with people who never mentioned the large chunk of food clearly stuck in my teeth, or how many times I have worked an entire work day without realizing my crazy eyebrows are making modern art and my ear hairs decided to grow an inch an hour. Indignities abound. In fact, the frequency, pace, and depth of these indignities only worsen with age.

It is important therefore to accept that this is a facet of life. It is a foundational pillar. Don't forget, you arrived all bloody, crying, and possibly having just sucked up muconium (baby poo) along the exit shute. Indiginities literally starts at the very beginning. And just like at the beginning, you were loved for just being you without any expectation that you would arrive clean, pure, and glowing – you should accept that aging is a process that has its own version of muconium all along the way. Your future as you age will not be different, no matter what great advice flows forth from this or any other book.

It is easier to unconditionally love others and yet the hardest thing in the world to love oneself unconditionally. I find that such a strange truism. If you are so lucky as to have a child or pet, you love them when they shit themselves or when they make the biggest mistakes of their lives and it will cost you hours and perhaps weeks of group suffering and possibly family therapy. You love them unconditionally because they simply are and they are yours and guess what, you simply are right now, too, and you are yours. But somehow when you were young, you internalized a whole array of expectations about yourself that were never realistic to start with but which serve as a barrier to fully loving yourself unconditionally, warts and all. Should your life always be awesome and you be perfect and glow all the time as the one exception on a planet of literally billions of people suffering indignities right now as we speak? No, it shouldn't and won't. You are exceptional but in this case not the exception. And that's fine, so long as you take a deep breath and accept reality as reality.

Now, remember your grandparents, if you were so blessed to have known them. Think about how you felt about them when you were young. You likely loved them unconditionally as well, even though they moved slower, were achy, forgot names, couch surfed to get to the kitchen table hobbling side to side, and wore adult diapers. You loved them because they simply were. Remember that as you age, because you simply are and you are simply not going to experience perfection and endlessly glow. In other words, to age well, you have to accept reality because to live in a myth is not going to serve you in any positive way. It will only deepen the hurt when life's muconium comes your way.

I have a phrase I have coined that I hope you will adopt. It is simply this: "More thrive-y." The goal in life is not to live a perfect life or to live to be perfect, but for you to endless strive to be more thrive-y.

"Thriving" is one of my favorite words. It is my goal for my patients, my children, my wife, my extended family members, and myself. It is a state of being where one is tapping into one's potential for feeling self-love, self-actuation, experiencing healthy connection with others, and feeling physically and emotionally prime. None of those are easy and rarely do all of these factors align perfectly to feel in a state as the psychologist Maslow called "self-actualized." If it is rare and not long lasting, feeling peak is hardly a good goal, as it is ephemeral – like a sugar high. Life is an endless juggling act of self, others, community, country, and humanity. Each of these get complicated quickly. It is easy to be beset by conflict and cacophony. Moments of harmony are wonderful but short lived.

If "peak" is not a great goal, then perhaps thriving is not such a great goal, given that often the two are confused with each other. Instead, the goal I share with you is not to thrive per say, but to work towards feeling more thrive-y. The goal is not an ideal state but the movement towards the ideal. Often it is said that: "it is the journey not the goal." In many ways, I am saying the same thing, except that I am being a bit more specific as to which journey. In this case, the journey is along a path of feeling physically thriving, emotionally thriving, unconditional self-loving, and connected with others in a more joyful and deeper manner. You don't ever have to get there. You just have to move the dial a tiny little bit more as time ticks forward.

Inn my faith we have a saying: you don't have to fix the world, you simply have to try (and preferably try your best). It is unacceptable to not try. But the burden of success is in no way on your shoulders. My goal of feeling more thrive-y is similar but is not a religious doctrine. There is no one asking you if you are thriving more today than you were yesterday and if not making a tsk tsk sound and looking at you dejectedly. If you are not more thrive-y today than you were yesterday, so be it. However, if you were more thrive-y today than yesterday, well that is something you can feel in your heart and enjoy all for yourself.

What does "more thrive-y" look like? It looks like eating a bit healthier today than yesterday, but not necessarily eating in some manner that is sold as "pure" or perfect. It looks like moving your body more today than you did yesterday, preferably more of your joints and perhaps a bit more cardio. It means reaching out to another person or more people and having more conversations, perhaps a bit more meatier and more meaningful than the weeks or months before, even if it is just one more person or one more question than you asked before. It means spending just a tiny bit more time in nature or in civic places. And mostly, it means doing this with absolutely no pressure on you, just the expression of a goal when it can be reached.

At its very center, more thrive-y has no purity, no perfection, no ideal. It is just a journey to enjoy and share. It is also a goal of this book. In addition to offering you utility, I also hope that it helps you feel more thrive-y today and perhaps also more thrive-y tomorrow. If it is making you feel more thrive-y a year from now, we should definitely plan a party.

Student Body

It is 1981. I am told that I need to write and re-write my letters in script. I write and re-write looping letters for what seems like eons every day. Apparently, my nine year old self has poor eye-hand coordination and my handwriting is atrocious (turns out, I have great hand-eye coordination, but my handwriting is just forever and all time atrocious – some would say I was meant to go into medicine).

It is 1986. I discover I have a photographic memory. For the next eight years, I take all of my tests in my minds eye revisiting where I wrote my notes, seeing every bored doodle exactly where I drew a face, a cockroach, or big circles around phrases. This is like finding out one has a super power but that it only works in stuffy classrooms with clocks that click like hammers hitting rock as the hands move slowly through each tired, sysophysian day. My super power doesn't get me dates or a starting position in my JV basketball team.

It is 1990. It doesn't matter that I am sick as a dog with what is likely Lyme Disease. I am enrolled in a college that produces the highest per capita PhDs in the United States and it is no challenge for my photographic mind at all. It is just a burdensome load of reading on top of the burden of chronic fatigue and the depression of a sometimes bedridden, once star athlete. Meanwhile, I meet students who have minds that don't even need to go to class and still destroy their exams. There are other super powers out there. I get some relief in knowing it scores no dates for them either.

It is 1999. I decide that I am such an outstanding student that I can take the Chinese acupuncture track, the Japanese acupuncture track, and the Chinese herbal medicine track at the oldest acupuncture school in the nation, where most students barely survive only one track. Some semesters, I am taking seven classes. I am passionate about the material and am a thirsty sponge.

It is 2024. My memory is for shit. I haven't had a photographic mind for decades now. But my memory is crap from Covid. I am fully functional on the outside, but internally I can tell something is very wrong. I feel like a super hero whose power is forcibly removed from them. I get my work done just fine but I am in psychic anxiety about my change of state. A discovery of mine leads me to supplement with DHEA. The difference is night and day. No photographic memory but now I am not forgetting what my wife just told me to grab at the supermarket 30 seconds earlier.

Each cell of the body is a student and life is the teacher. The cells – they are always learning their whole lives, adapting to life's blessings and curses. Adaptation is life and life is adaptation. This means for cells to survive, they have to be in constant communication with the world that they experience and adapt to changes in their environment. In many ways, this is the very reason why we have DNA – an encyclopedia of responses to life's glories and its cudgels.
As we get older, our cells simply do not adapt as readily and this is most clearly observable as a response to injury. Children heal like wildfire. As a healer, it is awe inspiring how quickly children bounce back. The opposite is true for people later in life – especially those in their fifties and beyond. It is less bouncing back and more doggedly and creakily chugging along. This is how injuries heal but you can imagine this is actually a greater issue affecting larger areas of the body – the speed of adaptation is greatly curtailed.

It is easy to blame this reduced adaptability and slower healing on "aging" as a general concept but instead I believe being specific is more powerful in identifying the cure. Inasmuch, we need to blame our students (our cells). Something has changed for them that has made them less responsive.

Imagine going to school and being told after the first 12 years of taking notes that today you get no pencil. Tomorrow, you get no paper. The next day, you have to plug one ear. The day after that, you must be blindfolded. It gets harder to learn the more impediments you add. The cells of our bodies have an accrued array of impediments – many of which I am going to discuss in this book. But there are two items I will discuss in this chapter that are very important.

The first one is DHEA. Think of DHEA like the paper you take your notes on. If you have no DHEA, you have to work around this impediment in order to learn. It would be a big blow to most students to not have a way to store memory by writing it down. Later in this book, I will talk about the importance of DHEA directly on memory as a whole (ie. remembering what you ate for dinner last night) but in the context of this conversation, I am talking about memory on a cellular level. Cells are receiving information from the tissues and fluids around them and then responding to these inputs by changing their state – akin to writing some notes in pencil on paper. At any point, the information might change and then you need to use the eraser on what you had inputted earlier and then write new notes about new exigent circumstances. DHEA allows you to be adaptable in this manner.

Cholesterol makes pregnenolone and pregnenolone converts into DHEA. How many people are on statins to reduce their cholesterol? And what does this mean for their pregnenolone? How does this impact their cellular memory via DHEA? I don't have an answer. I do, however, safely presume the elderly have always been slower to respond to new stimuli than the young. What is likely a bigger factor than statins reducing cholesterol in why our DHEA reduces over time is that certain fungi, which I am going to talk about in the next chapter in greater depth, dam up the pregnenolone and do not allow it to convert into anything else – especially DHEA. Other organisms also separately trick the body by producing the wrong shapes of DHEA so that it does not make enough of the proper, usable shapes of DHEA. No matter the mechanism, the net effect is low DHEA and this means on a cellular level, adaptation slows to a crawl. Cells stop responding effectively to their environmental inputs efficiently. In many ways, this is the epitome of aging.

As a practitioner of Chinese medicine, we do not believe in taking any food or supplement endlessly. We are not Western doctors who think you should stay on prescriptions for decades of life. Instead, we think you should use tools when you need them and then stop using them as soon as you don't. True, some Western medicines need to be used this way, but there are probably plenty that one could use episodically and this might prove to be more effective. Not my medicine, so not my fight. I do believe that episodic use of healing tools tends to be more powerful than constant use at least for much of what we do in Chinese medicine. This means the same tool will be just as strong when you need it again later and not weathered down by over use and perhaps the adaptation of other organisms to our treatment strategies. Which is to say, I absolutely do not believe and am in no way advocating that people should supplement DHEA endlessly from the day they turn 50 to the day they die. What I am suggesting to my readers is that when you have a new issue that has arisen and your healing response is slower than expected, no matter what the issue is, take DHEA for the next month (or until it makes you feel brooding and angstful) as you continue your healing strategies – no matter how, with what modality, and with what mechanism you approach your healing. In other words, this is a general rule to apply. In programmer language: "IF new problem arises and it doesn't go away as quickly as expected THEN take DHEA for a month as one tries to heal it through any healing tool or medicine." The exception to this is if your Western medical practitioner feels this is not a safe strategy for you.

For instance, if you test high for DHEA in blood tests, this might not be right for you. If you have high androstendione (which DHEA converts into) or high testosterone in blood tests, this strategy might not be right for you. But for most aging people, these are not likely issues specifically because the DHEA is already low and therefore everything downstream hormonally in the cascade of how one hormone makes another is lower as well.

The second important factor for the adaptability of cells unfortunately is something that I am only learning about now, 25 years into my career: the importance of peptides in turning genes on and off. In my student years, I took microbiology and even classes on genetics. I spent a Summer as a DNA testing specialist in a white coat lab full of fun glass vials and test tubes. Never once did we learn there is a major groove and a minor groove in the double helix DNA strands where peptides land and in doing so play a role in activating or inhibiting gene expression. I pride myself in still learning something new every day and it was my 25th year in medicine when I learned this.

Different peptides activate or inhibit different genes. They are gene specific. This is, in many ways, a very important part of the adaptation on a cellular level to environmental factors. This also means an accruel of chronic infections as one gets older and older often results in an excessive overload of pathogen toxin versions of peptides, which no doubt plays a nasty, additive role in reducing cell adaptability. As of this writing, I am doing my own professional deep dive into better understanding how to interact with this molecular phenomenon. In much of the book, I will make many assertions that are based on decades of hard work but I do have to admit when and where I am a beginner to honestly represent myself and as peptides go, I am a newborn. I have a list of about 220 peptides I am feverishly investigating. I can absolutely see that this work is very important but it might be future editions of this book where I can offer better self-care ideas for clearing pathogen peptides. In the meantime, I offer you a wide array of thoughtful strategies to help you avoid chronic infections that effect aging and no doubt these organisms that are avoided through these strategies are ones that would play some negative role in regards to pathogen toxin peptides. In other words, the best I can offer you today is preventative medicine, which you will find especially in the chapter at the end of the book about a calendar for effective self-care.

Key Takeways:

- If you have a new symptom and it doesn't go away quickly, go on DHEA supplementation for a month (or until it makes you feel brooding or angstful) each time this happens. This possibly won't help, but improving cellular adaptability is giving yourself the best chance to speed up recovery

A Very Fungal Problem

It is 1991. I am visiting my one day wife, my one day brother-in-law, and my one day in-laws at their house for the first time. They live in an old 1800s farm house in coastal Maine, not far from where a tidal river meets the ocean. The nature outside is verdant and road trips are majestic, hilly, and bump against a sprawling ocean shoreline that can take your breath away, especially if you have a photographer's eye.

I have been in their house for four hours. The coughing has begun. I have been in their house for eight hours. The taste of blood is now palpable with every cough. It is the next day and fatigue joins the cough. I feel frustrated and sour. I am now a week out from my visit to their house, and my cut up lungs are still recovering with a persisting cough. It goes on and on.

Repeat this cycle twice a year for decades.

I am now a medical intuitive. I have figured it out. I am exposed to Alternaria, a tree fungus, in their house which is heated by a wood stove. It isn't their house that wants to kill me (my long held suspicion), it is the fungus that wants to colonize me. It is producing estrogens and progesterones in my lungs to cause swelling and a cough. It is producing serotonins that are swimming in my blood that causes a foul mood and massive frustration. It is producing cortisol that is making me exhausted.

Before you start this chapter, if you are a germaphobe – have a real genuine phobia about germs, you probably should skip most of this chapter and jump to the "What Can I Do?" section below. In fact, much of this book is about the influence of microbes on our bodies. My goal is not to increase any latent fears one might have about microbes but for us all to better understand how to live in balance in vast complex ecosystems around us and in us with healthy habits. Human bodies are ecosystems and this is a good thing. It should be our goal to promote our bodies to be lush and verdant rain forests, helping to protect ourselves from developing monoculture (metaphorically speaking) anywhere in our bodies (which is arguably the goal of most infectious diseases). The healthier the flora natural to your system, the less likely you will be susceptible to infections. So, if you are a germaphobe, I encourage you to see yourself as the rain forest and that the germs to be frightened of are the ones that would want to plough down the ecosystem for their own profit.

Our nails are amazing. They are not quite bone – hard but pliable and tightly bound to the fingers and toes. Unfortunately, they are also incompletely bound, which means there are gaps between the nail beds and nails. Furthermore, we are sticking our fingers into all kinds of weird things over the course of hours, days, weeks, months, and years. Our toes are also close to the ground with all of the life that lives in the soil. The microbial soup of our environment normally is repelled by skin but when it comes to nails, it can get nicely wedged in, where over time fungal organisms protected from hand washing and other environmental factors can eventually colonize cuticles that are rich in capillaries and blood vessels, becoming a grapple hold for what will unfortunately become lifelong infections. The nails are usually the first location of assault by fungus for all humans except perhaps those living in the most arid deserts on the planet. Which is to say, practically all humans have fungal colonies in cuticles within the first few years of life that will bombard them internally with spores endlessly for decades upon decades to come. There are also other vectors of human infection: lungs, upper airways, ears, and eyes also lend themselves to what we in Chinese medicine call "pernicious forces"…or infectious "pathogens." Pathogens are the generic term for infectious organisms in Chinese medicine.

The term "pernicious" comes from the classics of Chinese medicine that are thousands of years old. This phrase is particularly apt for fungi. Unlike viruses and bacteria that cannot help but cause massive destruction in the wake of their infections that all but screams "I am infecting you right now," fungi are the total opposite. These organisms are stealthy, slow, methodical, and persistent. They are so stealthy that the Western medical world barely recognizes these organisms as infectious with few internal fungal infections in their diagnostic paradigm outside of dermatological disorders. In Chinese medicine, however, this is quite the opposite.

Fungi are a form of what we call "Damp Pathogens" which means they live in Damp environments. Notice the word Damp has a capital "D" which is to emphasize that I am making reference to the Chinese medical term of Dampness and not colloquial "dampness" meaning dank or wet. Dank or wet environments also happen to be Damp but Dampness is a much larger subject with broader connotations. As mentioned in the chapter on "Dying," you can broadly interpret Dampness as low oxygen environments in the body.

Unlike viruses and bacteria which live or die based on the environment immediately available to them, fungi generate their ideal environments around them wherever they grow. Like humans, they build their own version of huts, apartments, McMansions, and town houses as their colonies grow. And what I mean by this is that they are so good at constructing the ideal environment for their longevity, if a person takes an anti-fungal and it wipes out the current colony, all it takes is a new exposure with a fresh batch of fungus with access to the cities and towns made by previous generations and in short order the new colony can be back to the previous colony's size. It might have taken decades to slowly build their infrastructure but once it is there, the speed of reinfection is a hundred times faster. Anyone who has had a recurring experience with Candida yeast will recognize exactly what I am saying. It may sound like a contradiction, but fungi can be easy to clear but almost impossible to eradicate. It has to do with their houses. It has to do with low oxygen environments. It also has to do with pathogens being far far far more complex than humans realize.

Dampness is a common diagnosis in Chinese medicine. We tend to associate it with stagnant problems, hard to clear that can last months, years, and even decades. The energy no longer moves smoothly and gets easily stuck. Dampness tends to also associate with pain. Stagnation, persistent problems, stuck muscles/tendons/ligaments, and pain all sound familiar as a facet of the aging process, doesn't it? Which is to say, the number one focus you should have in aging comfortably is not just clearing fungus but ***regularly*** clearing fungus, preferably every three to four months. The need for regular clearing is two fold: 1. You are always exposed to fungi via spores in the air, in our clothes, in nail cuticles, and also via food and water. 2. And, as I said, it is easier to clear the colonies than to remove the cities they created within you, which means their colonies can rebound in size within months. And you should adapt to this knowledge with a change in strategy. Know they will rebound, prepare for this, and execute a habituated response.

There are many species of fungi (millions upon millions actually) and these species hybridize easily with other organisms to create new variants, making the spectrum of their variety practically endless. That said, there are certain strains that are more common than others in our human abodes, our food supply, and our external environments: Stachybotrys, Alternaria, Aspergillus, Fusarium, Penicillium, and yeasts of all sorts (Candida often becoming a stand-in name for what are actually quite a wide variety of non-Candida yeasts). Furthermore, all fungi in one's diet can be infectious as well including cooking yeasts, wine yeasts, nutritional yeast, and mushrooms.

There is a whole food industry out there telling you yeasts and mushrooms are ideal for diet, beneficial in innumerable ways such as sources of proteins, bioflavanoids, and more. There are also millions of species of fungi and no doubt there are medicinal and biologically beneficial factors and facets to fungi and yeasts. There are whole books on the subject by practitioners and healers of all sorts. I don't dispute any of this. There are good things in yeasts, fungi, and mushrooms. But, as someone who spends all day long clearing infections from people as I closely watch the aging process, I perceive quite a lot of harm caused by these organisms. I am personally not risking it. I avoid mushrooms in my diet even if they are considered excellent sources of protein. I avoid nutritional yeast and yeast additives as much as possible. I do, however, eat bread and so I know there are yeasts introduced regularly if not daily into my body. It is a data point for me and a reminder to do my regular maintenance care of clearing fungi every quarter. As I said, I am not trying to live a "pure" life. I am trying to live a high quality one. If you are a die hard yeast and mushroom enthusiast and will continue to eat these no matter what I write here, I encourage you to clear fungus from your system not once every three or four months but monthly instead. Which is to say, adapt my rules to your circumstance. Don't just say "Ethan hates mushrooms so he is an idiot and I reject all of his ideas." Rather, accept your personal inclination to eat fungal foods and adjust your strategy accordingly. It will make a big difference.

When I say fungi and yeast are infectious, I mean to say these organisms are perhaps the greatest negative influences in your life. Period. Of course, everyone is different and facing different circumstances, but for most people what I just wrote is exactly true. They are quiet, stealthy, and absolutely terrible. Here is just one example. Fungi swim in circulation waiting for you to injure yourself, at which point they will infect real estate in the body they could not previously reach, slowing down the healing process from injuries and surgeries often by adding weeks and months to recoveries. Here is another: most pains you have had in your life come from Dampness and Damp pathogens – and most Damp pathogens are fungal. Which means most pains in your life (especially arthritic ones) are from fungal sources.

As an aside, you may not know that anaerobic varieties of fungi often produce little hairy threads called mycelium. Mycelium are a network of vessels for the transport of nutrients but they also work like threads akin to the threads that construct your clothes. Anaerobic fungi also like to live in our bodies and they grow these same structures inside of us, which cause worsening mobility over time – joints that bend less and less every year. So not only do fungi cause arthritis, they also cause worsening flexibility and greater tightness of our soft tissues and joints over time.

It is very common for my patients who go on gluten free and sugar free diets to have major positive changes in energy, vitality, remarkable weight loss, and body comfort. I personally do not eat this way, but I see this as a consistent pattern. One very big reason for this is that sugar feeds fungi and yeast and commonly there is yeast in foods with gluten. Such a diet helps to kill off these colonies that have relied heavily on one's sugar intake to grow. The subsequent improvement in life force and vitality is palpable. You certainly could elect to remove these from your diet and if it is not a tall order for you, I encourage it. For me, it is a step too far as I get most of my life's enjoyment from food. I simply try to eat as low sugar as I can tolerate, knowing it will fuel all kinds of microbial activity inside my system.

Here are some common issues that arise with specific yeast

species:

- Stachybotrys – bone spurs, poor detoxing, anger, and fatigue
- Aspergillus – any health complaint with low dopamine (ie. Parkinson's, depression, Alzheimer's, and more), arthritis, estrogen and progesterone imbalances, chronic sinusitis, fatigue
- Alternaria – major bone swelling forms of arthritis, asthma, estrogen and progesterone imbalances, chronic swelling, chronic sinusitis, fatigue
- Fusarium – poor detoxing
- Penicillium – "auto-immune" complaints
- Yeast – vaginitis, urinary tract infections, bloating, acne, chronic sinusitis

These are only meant to be quick to digest examples. However, it is my belief that fungi are a fuel for most of the more complex diseases we develop over time in our lives – of which there are innumerable across every domain of medicine – urological, reproductive, ear/nose/throat, immunology, and more. This is why I tell everyone, if you want to age with the least amount of suffering, you absolutely must clear fungus every three to four months because the preventative value is incalcable.

Now, I do want to counsel you that there are many paths to Rome. Any one disease can have multiple possible causes. Desulfavibrio is a non-fungal pathogen that also causes dopamine issues, by way of example. Bacillus Thuringiensis, a common soil bacteria, also causes major estrogen and progesterone imbalances. Staphylococcus species can wear down cartilage and cause bone-on-bone arthritis. You will not find me in the "fungus causes every problem known to man" camp. However, if you regularly clear fungus from the body, you are taking away additional fuel to the fire that can lead down these avenues and more.

Fungal pathogens are the original endocronologists but in reverse: evil geniuses. Over the span of billions of years, they have figured out how to generate hormones. Not every infectious organism has developed this technological know-how. A very important thing you absolutely need to understand is this: your hormones are your emotions. This means that fungi and yeasts play us like puppets, pulling our emotional heartstrings in ways that best serves them. You think it is a coincidence you have bloating but feel sad and crave ice cream? No, that yeast producing the gas in your abdomen is also boosting sugar cravings and convincing you that you need to self-nurture away your sadness and frustration. Just think of the incredibly complex nature of such subterfuge. Not only has it infected your body, found safe places to form colonies sizable enough for its off-gassing to distend your abdomen, it boosts ghrelin, a hunger hormone, and serotonin, a mood altering hormone, in order to convince your body it should eat more foods that it specifically wants (fast sugars) to feed its growth. If it wasn't terrible, it would be miraculous, honestly. But it is terrible because it means fungal pathogens have a complex understanding of how to manipulate their hosts to change their habits and activities to suit their needs. These are microbial gaslighters.

As I said, I recommend regularly clearing fungi and yeast from your system. Each time you do this, you will likely experience a process known as a Herxheimer Reaction. Your lymphatic system is a highway for white blood cells. When fungi or other organisms die and release the toxins inside of them, your white blood cells are charged with cleaning up the debris field left behind. A small amount of fungus means a small amount of clean up whereas a large amount means a large many white blood cells are needed to perform widescale cleaning. Whenever white blood cells clean an area, the lymphatic system temporarily becomes stagnant in that location. This can lead to achiness, a foggy head, fatigue, and/or irritability – which is the Herxheimer Reaction. The way to minimize this is to keep your lymphatic system flush. Your stomach will turn plain water (nothing at all added, not even lemon juice) into lymphatic fluid. Therefore, when you are clearing fungus and for the next few days, it is ideal to drink no less than 5 cups of plain water a day, each 8 ounces at a minimum, to keep your lymphatic fluid flush.

What Can I Do?

To kill off yeast, you can employ the same recommendations from the earlier chapter titled "Dying" where I spoke about anaerobic pathogens. You can use hyperbaric oxygen chambers twice a week for two weeks (a bit faster of a schedule than to kill off anaerobes to accommodate for the fact fungi and yeast will replicate faster than anaerobes) or three cups a day of nettle tea for two weeks. You can also make use of other interventions such as Caprylic Acid tinctures (follow the instructions on the bottle), oregano oil drops 7 drops a day morning and evening for one week (not everyone can tolerate this oil as it is very strong – I, for one, break out in rashes with it), and direct treatment of skin and nail infections with apple cider finger soaks or creams with tea tree oil.

Nails are the locations of the oldest colonies and are therefore the hardest to clear of fungus. You may spend your whole life trying and never clear them, unfortunately. There are some unpleasant truths in this book and one of them is that not every infection can be 100% cleared. You will never be 100% fungus free and that should not be your goal. Your goal should be to keep any such colonies in check, with limited colonies in limited places and therefore limited influence on your health and well being.

As an aside, I will note that super thick nails is not always a sign of fungus. If the nail is very thick (ie. more than 2 mm), it is actually more likely to be HPV virus infecting the cuticle, causing an overproduction of keratin, collagen, fibrin, and elastin. Another hard truth: being that HPV is a viral issue, there is even less you can do to clear it with home remedies, unfortunately.

Mildew, Algae, Moss, and Lichen

Only in recent months, have I come to discover that mildews infect the body. I have known that algae, moss, and lichen can infect as well but never realized mildew could pose a serious health challenge until my 25th year in practice – and only gave sparse attention to these other pathogens. You won't hear any doctors of any medicine diagnose you with a mildew or lichen infection – and that is looking increasingly misguided. One reason for this is that I feel these pathogens primarily infect in super tiny sizes of scale (nanos). My clinical focus has thus far been tilted heavily towards yeast and fungi on the topic of what we call "Damp Pathogens" in Chinese medicine. It very much looks like these other organisms are just as problematic as the primary focus of my antagonism. For instance, blood pressure issues, urinary and bowel incontinence issues, and cataracts may all potentially associate with these "unusual" infections (if they cause any of these common issues, how "unusual" are they really?). I do not as yet have the level of confidence to proclaim these or any assertions boldly. Future versions of this book will wax eloquent on the nasty impacts of these microbes. But, alas, the current state of my knowledge about what these do in the body and which remedies help to effectively clear them is unfortunately limited at the time of this writing.

Key Takeaways:

- Fungal pathogens are the major cause of pain and limitation of movement in the body. They also negatively impact our emotional state to manipulate us for their benefit
- Like anaerobes, fungal pathogens (some of which are anaerobic) need a low oxygen environment in which to live
- Clearing fungal pathogens every three to four months is the most important preventative care you can employ to age more comfortably and more gracefully
- Stay tuned for future versions of this book where I discuss mildew, algae, moss, and lichen with more experience and more confidence

Bone Softening

It is 1977. I am five years old. My grandmother just passed away at a shocking young age. We are in the limousine leaving the funeral home on our way to the cemetery where I will soon see my father cry for the first time. I am sitting with my grandfather who just lost the love of his life. He will die soon thereafter from a broken heart.

As a toddler, I am mesmerized by my grandfather's elbows. The skin is so droopy – nothing like my youthful, taut skin. I squeeze his extra, dangling elbow skin and I say loudly and unselfconsciously: "pinchy winchy winchy." It temporarily breaks the somber moment and the car erupts with smiles and laughter, a moment of levity like a camera flash quickly cutting the darkness.

The droopy skin of our aging process that announces to one and all that we are no longer emissaries of youth has a cause and the cause and it is not collagen, elastin, or fibrin – the basis of most self-care cures for rejuvenation. Instead, the cause is much deeper: our bones. Our bones are an infrastructure upon which softer tissues of our bodies gain some amount of anchor and purchase. As we age, our bones soften and lose mass sometimes quickly but mostly slowly. You can think of this akin to a subtle melting that takes years and decades to degrade enough for the soft tissues around the bone to sag like balloons slowly deflating.

In many ways, our bones are the most important tissues of our bodies. In Chinese medicine, they are the coldest tissue, comprised of Water Qi, the coldest of the Five Elements. Water Qi is controlled by Earth Qi and life is lived in an Earth Qi environment not because we live on "planet Earth" but because our sun is a purveyor of Earth Qi, constantly embracing us with Earth Qi every day our whole lives. As a result, our bones eventually are "controlled" (from a Five Element perspective on how one Element controls another Element) more and more as the years add up, melting subtly along the way.

You can think of bones akin to a refrigerator. Being the coldest tissue of the body, they cool down our softer tissues akin to a refrigerator cooling down the food within it. In both cases, the cooling effect discourages the growth of pathogens. Turn off your refrigerator for only a few hours and mold will quickly expand its colonies all over your apples, cheese, and broccoli. Same with our soft tissues – if the bones warm up too much, the local soft tissues experience an increased risk of infection. Our lives are lived in a microbial soup and we are bombarded daily by micro-organisms. It doesn't take long for infections in the body to spread and deepen in areas around warm bones. This occurs at the same time of life when blood vessels are more clogged with plaque and scar tissues, bone marrow is less productive in making white blood cells, and the lymphatic system is less fully functional as a highway for the white blood cells. Younger people experience infections in a more pronounced manner because their systems are more efficient at recognizing a problem and mounting a counter-attack. But at an older age, we experience chronic infections with fewer warning signs due to ever increasing inefficiencies building up throughout the system.

Healthy, full bones means aging with more taut, youthful looking skin, fewer chronic infections, and therefore more vitality. The more infections sprouting up around the body quietly, the less energy, stamina, and vigor. This is why I say the bones are the most important tissue to protect as you age – certainly not for the aesthetic value of taut skin, but because once chronic infections set in, problems multiply.

Unfortunately, just taking bone boosting minerals regularly (which is a good idea) is not enough. Instead, you have to identify warning signs and address them as they arise in order to best guard your system and protect your life force.

Arthritis

At this stage of my career, I am aware of three factors that generate arthritis: fungal infections, Staphylococcus sub variants (specifically MRSA and MRCONs), and Bacillus Thuringiensis (a common soil bacteria).

The previous chapter was all about fungus and its negative influence in our lives. Chronic fungal infections are the most common cause of arthritis and body pains. Please see that chapter for a detailed analysis.

Staphylococcus causes a very specific type of arthritis: rapid destruction of cartilage in joints leading to "bone-on-bone" disorders and often the need for joint replacements. Despite autoclaving and other "clean room" measures, I have found that most surgeries come with an uninvited exposure to these Staphylococcus variants. This means that surgeries today can lead to joint replacements tomorrow, metaphorically speaking. The best way to avoid this and also to address any latent Staphylococcus in the body is to to take Goldenseal herb 1000mg twice daily for a week following every Western intervention in which the skin is broken or intubation or catherization is required. Alternatively, liquid colloidal silver can be used 1 teaspoon twice a day for five days. MRSA and MRCONs are notoriously resistant to antibiotics. The best tool to clear it is actually Manuka honey from New Zealand as it is replete with anti-microbial molecules. Studies have demonstrated it maintains effectiveness regardless of the resistance level of the pathogen. Unfortunately, Manuka is best for infections that can be treated topically (you can put Manuka directly into open wounds), but most surgical exposures spread these pathogens far from the original sites of exposure such as surgical wounds or the airway. This means, the best tools are systemic ones such as Goldenseal and colloidal silver. Homeopaths might have what are called "nosodes" for these pathogens, which might be a worthy intervention to explore. But I have no experience using these with my patients.

Bacillus Thuringiensis is a bacterial pathogen that can generate hot hormones similar to fungus, leading to chronic swelling known as edema. This can occur in blood vessels, lymphatic vessels, bone surface tissues (called periosteum), and more, as a contributor to arthritis. As these are bacterial in nature, the same recommendations for Goldenseal and colloidal silver apply, however, I would recommend once every three months applying these for one week to help reduce any resident colonies.

Gardeners should consider applying these methods once a month instead of once a quarter during gardening seasons, as your exposure is much higher.

As an aside, pathogens have many ways that they hide in the body in dormant or protected states that can make it very hard to fully eradicate infections once they have become resident. While my own treatment methods account for this, tools such as Goldenseal and colloidal silver can only eradicate what is immediately accessible to them – which means active infections. This is why regular application of these tools are necessary, because you can only clear what is active while the potential energy (dormant, hidden varieties) remains untouched and the infections will return eventually over time.

Osteopenia/Osteoporosis

Everyone experiences bone loss as we age as a facet of living within an energy system in which we are daily exposed to the power and influence of the Sun. As I said, the Sun generates Earth Qi, the energy that controls the Water Qi in the bones, which means over time, it can melt our bones. That said, some people obviously experience bone loss faster than others and receive a diagnosis of osteopenia at the onset of a degenerative process that at later stages is known as osteoporosis.

These are very real biological processes, but what is often lost in the conversation is the fact that symptoms often come on in a very short period of time going from doing just fine to suddenly having major, problematic skeletal issues (ie. bone fractures). What accounts for this? From a Western perspective, there are two triggers of note: genetics and menopause. Diet should also be added as a factor, but is often overlooked by physicians.

However, there are two contributing factors that are entirely unrelated to genetics, diet, and menopause that are entirely within your radius of control that are actually major factors that are completely invisible to Western consideration. Forgive me, they are gross. But let's face these factors together: mites and pinworms.

In fact, we do face these factors together because at any given moment in time, it is thought that more than 11% of the human population has pinworm in them. It is a shockingly successful organism and is equally problematic across all socio-economic levels, which means it is not an issue of poverty or poor access to regular hygiene. It is very likely that you, as a reader of this book, have pinworm in you. In fact, I would say the likelihood it is in you is probably closer to 100% but the probability that it is active and and an issue is closer to 5-10%. What does that mean? As I said, we live in a microbial soup. We are exposed daily to organisms in the air, our food supply, our home environments, our family members, friends, and community, plus other vectors of exposure – and yet we are not massive biological messes. Even the weakest, most frail, and most vulnerable among us have powerful immune systems that keep the vast majority of infectious organisms under control. You likely have pinworm and a whole host of other organisms within the bounds of your body but the environment must be "just right" for these opportunistic organisms to flourish, since most of the time your immune system is kicking ass and taking names.

Pinworm, like most organisms, attack people as members of larger groups of organisms called "colonies." This is not known to Western medicine and yet it is so obvious once you look for it. This is the major reason why infections are hard to clear once resident – most infectious organisms work together as teams that keep each other alive. Different organisms survive in different internal biomes within the body such that if you successfully clear pathogens from one biome, if a member of the colony can persist in another biome, the entire colony has a good chance of surviving and eventually resurging – for instance in moist versus dry locations of the body. Most people suffer recurring infections as a consequence of this fact. You have to attack all organisms in the colony to generate a robust and permanent healing. Pinworms always live in a colony with Candida, Entamoeba, and Gardnerella. You may recognize some of these organisms as common factors in vaginitis.

Back to the original question: Why is pinworm a factor for osteopenia and/or osteoporosis? Pinworm, if it is growing in the body, causes malabsorption of vitamins and minerals. It literally steals the minerals from your food and supplements and uses this to fuel its own growth. This will show up often with an associated symptom of fatigue as these minerals and vitamins are important for your vitality. This malabsorption affects many tissues but it is most obvious in the bones because when bones don't have the minerals they need, they become brittle. The risk for bone associated symptoms such as fractures rises tremendously. Bone pains that won't go away may be a sign of a chip in a bone that does not have enough minerals accessible to it in order to fully heal. Teeth can chip. To me, a broken bone especially from a minor insult is a warning sign of a mineral malabsorption issue and therefore pinworm has to be assessed.

But pinworm is not the only organism that causes mineral malabsorption and so the list of suspects is a bit larger. We must also suspect mites. We all have tiny little creatures called mites that live on and even in our bodies. To the most part, I tell people it is fine to know about these little dudes but probably better not to think too much about them because, yes, it is yucky. Demodex mites are the most common variety of mite on and in us. Demodex mites live in our hair follicles and serve an important role in our ecosystem by eating up dead cells as they flake off. But Demodex mites are not the only kind of mite that can live off the human body. There is actually a wide array of mites that include wood mites, dust mites, bird mites, flour mites, and more that can survive on and even in our bodies. To the most part, we are in symbiosis with these mites. We need those dead cells to go and new ones to take their place. However, there are circumstances in which these mites over-populate. When they do this, they cause mineral malabsorption just as problematic as pinworm if not more so and the result is the same array of skeletal complaints.

In Chinese medicine, every human being has an energy "constitution" that determines your fundamental strengths and weaknesses. Furthermore, we live in a complex interplay with energy cycles that are as short as every 15 minutes and as long as every 60 years. Each year of this 60 year cycle, there are two energies that are active during that year (the energies change every year at Chinese New Year – which is why it is the "New Year"). As I write this book, the current year energies are Water Qi and Earth Qi year, a combination that clearly fuels the growth of mite populations as my patients have been inundated with mite overgrowth all Summer long. Fatigue, fractures, and new diagnosis of osteopenia and osteoporosis has dotted the Summer among this population. Which is to say, prevention for mites is all but impossible because you cannot change what fuels their growth as these cycles are literally conscribed by the movements of the planets in our solar system (the movement of these planets determine the two energies active each year). Another sign of mites being more active is random itching around the body, hives, and rashes.

If you suspect pinworm, you might bring this up to your primary care physician. There are over-the-counter remedies for this that are very mild but they might not be right for you based on your unique physiology, prescribed medications, and circumstances. However, taking an over-the-counter remedy is not enough, since it exists within a colony. As mentioned earlier, pinworm lives in a colony that includes a yeast, an amoeba, and a bacteria. If you have ever experienced Candiditis, you know it is very hard to remedy this situation by just taking anti-fungals alone such as Nystatin or Diflucan. The reason for this is the same reason – Candida exists in a colony with these other organisms that protect its survival. This means, to work on pinworm, you must approach this with a multi-pronged approach that addresses parasites, yeast, and bacteria. The long way to do this is to go off sugar for three to six months to rob these organisms of fuel they use to thrive. But there are faster ways. For bacteria, you can use those same tools mentioned earlier: Goldenseal and colloidal silver, taking these for two weeks rather than one week. At the same time, you need to take natural anti-parasitics such as black walnut and wormwood, taking these for a month following the directions on their packaging. For Candida, you must treat this with anti-fungals such as 7 drops of Oil of Oregano in ¼ cup water twice a day for two weeks or caprylic acid according to the directions on the bottle for two weeks. And yes, follow the same recommendations if you have been having chronic, recurring yeast infections and also urinary tract infections, as these same pathogens may be playing a role in these situations as well.

Mites are a more complex issue to address via self-care, as to the most part, you can consider these organisms part of the microbiome but which has grown beyond healthy bounds. Yes, mites also live in colonies, but in this case, they are the top of what I call a "Life Cycle" – which means there are numerous organisms that infect the body with the main goal of ultimately engendering mites in the ecosystem – too many organisms to address as a strategy. There are insecticides that kill mites but layering your body with insecticide is not high on the list of strategies you will find a Chinese medical practitioner promoting. Tea tree oil is a potent insecticide and can be used in cream form to cover the body. One can become sensitive to tea tree oil and it is important to avoid using this strategy too often. However, if you use this approach once in a blue moon, put 10 drops of tea tree oil in a carrier oil or cream and wipe this on all skin surfaces. Leave it there for an hour then wash it off. Sulfur kills mites, and so bathing in sulfur hotsprings is a good strategy if that is available to you. Apple cider vinegar can be wiped on the skin and left there for an hour then washed off. I would recommend not applying this on all skin surfaces all at once but instead applying this to arms, legs, torso, and face at separate times of the day to avoid overwhelming your system with the vinegar.

There is another contributing factor for osteopenia and osteoporosis that I haven't yet mentioned as it does not rob your body of minerals but instead tricks your body into not making new bone. Bone is living tissue and is constantly cycling through a process of breaking down bone where you do not need it and building new bone where you need it more. This is hugely adaptive as it means that you might live a life that is not very physical and you need less bone to accomplish your acts of daily living but you can change vocations and suddenly be in a physically demanding job and your bones will literally grow to accommodate your changing needs.

Clostridium Difficile is a pathogen known to most people as a diarrhea bug one might catch in a hospital that is very difficult to eradicate. But the truth is that it is much more prevalent than that. We all have some of this pathogen in our bodies and most of us do not suffer diarrhea, which is to say it has other locations of the body where it can thrive. Unfortunately, one such location is in bone cells called osteoblasts. We have two main bone cells: osteocytes that break down bone and osteoblasts that build new bone. If you have a pathogen such as Clostridium Difficile selectively infecting osteoblasts while leaving osteocytes alone, you have a recipe for reducing bone without building it back up. This is another pathway for more bone loss over time, albeit a slower path towards osteopenia and osteoporosis than the previously mentioned parasitic pathways. If you are experiencing a very slow drift towards osteoporosis, this might be the more likely vector.

Clostridium Difficile can attack alone or in colonies with other organisms. Despite it co-infecting with the pandemic Coronavirus Sars-CoV-2, I do not have a strong grock on other common co-infectors at this moment in time. The good news, however, is that Clostridium species are anaerobic and this means our same oxygen building tools discussed earlier in the book (nettle tea and hyperbaric oxygen chambers) are great choices. However, given the fact that these are internal infections to cells, once every two months is likely to be more protective than once a quarter in slowing down osteopenia.

Cadmium Deficiency

Cadmium is an often maligned ingredient of life and there is a reason for it. You can think of it akin to a cellular battery pack. Virtually every cell needs this battery pack to function. Too many batteries, however, will cause a cell to become hyperactive. This can lead to allergies and auto-immune activity when the microbiome and white blood cells absorb too much cadmium. However, on the opposite side of the equation, too little cadmium means not enough energy inside the cell to reach peak cellular performance. This becomes a problem in cells such as osteoblasts that build bone and chondrocytes that build cartilage. Under performance of these cells means bone and cartilage tissues are not constructed. This is another pathway to develop bone loss and cartilage loss over time, as these are tissues that need regular reconstruction.

At this moment in time, I do not recommend cadmium supplementation because the system is simply too sensitive to cadmium. Some cells will absorb too much and become hyperactive in a terrible way. Getting it to the exact cells that need it while avoiding those that don't is effectively impossible.

Softening Bones

There is a molecule in bones that makes bones physically hard that organisms sometimes steal and replace with the mirror image molecule that is also bonded to a metal (known as a chelated isomer) that consequently softens bones. This essential molecule is called 21-deoxycortisol. When the chelated isomer of 21-deoxycortisol builds up in a bone or tooth, what should be hard loses that super power, which brings us to the title of this chapter. The softening of bone and teeth is unfortunately a common phenomenon. Similar to osteoporosis and osteopenia, this increases the risk of bone chipping and fracturing but it also increases the likelihood of joint pain. Bones are meant to be hard but when they are soft and pliable, the mechanical nature of joints breaks down. Imagine gears of a clock where the gears are soft rather than hard. In no time, this will gum up the operation of the clock. First, those gears will work less efficiently; eventually the gears will simply stop. Unlike a clock, however, our bodies are filled with nerves that do not respond well to unexpected increases in stimulation. Softening bones means more surface areas touch each other longer than expected and this is therefore a pathway to pain.

Is this arthritis? Arguably. But arguably this is a different but similar phenomenon in which joints get sticky and inefficient.

There are two organisms that produce this phenomenon I will mention in this section and another one I will mention in the next section. Staphylococcus (especially MRSA and MRCONs) and Bacillus Thuringiensis, two of our three main antagonists for arthritis, produce the toxins that cause this softening. Please see strategies noted earlier in how to clear these.

Outside of my methodology, I do not know how to clear the chelated isomers of 21-deoxycortisol once it has infiltrated the bone and teeth tissues. As far as I know, there are also no supplements specific to this hardly known cortisol subtype. This leaves us in a pickle in terms of self-care. At the very least, I recommend following the anti-bacterial protocols mentioned earlier in this chapter. This should slow down the softening process. I also recommend switching toothpastes from the regular varieties sold in every day pharmacies to ones that remineralize the teeth with hydroxyapetite crystals, as these toothpastes provide additional firmness to the teeth enamel. This is a strategy you should definitely employ if you have started to experience chips in your teeth. The toothpaste does not provide any benefit to bone and will not do anything beneficial in the case of jaw bone degeneration, however. But it can reverse softening of the teeth.

Rapid Bone Loss And/Or Teeth Degradation

There are pathogens in every human body that can proliferate under the right circumstances that can cause rapid bone loss at specific joints (rather than whole body) and can cause massive teeth erosion. You can see this most easily when looking at the teeth of dogs. One day they may look fine, but the next day, the teeth may have turned a dark color and suddenly half a tooth has crumbled away. People with poor dental hygiene are more prone to seeing this same phenomenon with their teeth. But even people with fine dental hygiene can find themselves suddenly having a sudden abscess from the same phenomenon.

The problem has a name that we have all heard of but none of us think is relevant to every day humans living every day lives: gangrene….or, more specifically Clostridium Perfringins, the organism that causes gangrene. Gangrene is the phenomenon that Clostridium Perfringins causes. Clostidium Perfringens causes massive, rapid bone and teeth degeneration by softening these tissues so quickly and so tremendously that the bone simply can't hold itself together. Which is to say, it is the same chelated isomers of 21-deoxycortisol that cause this phenomenon, but C. Perfringens is an organism on steroids (metaphorically speaking) when it is active.

Clostridium Perfringens increases its activity in our bodies as we age. It does this because as we age we develop worse circulation plus more scar tissue and this is an anaerobic bacteria, which means it requires low oxygen environments in which to thrive. Once again, I recommend nettle tea and hyperbaric oxygen chambers as strategies for reducing anaerobic pathogens in the body (see the previous chapter *A Very Fungal Problem* for detailed recommendations). As you can see, it is very important for multiple reasons to clear anaerobic pathogens from your body every three to four months.

Microtubules And Microfilaments

Our bodies are constructed out of blueprints that we generally associate with genes and DNA. However, this is not entirely correct. Genes produce proteins and proteins construct our bodies. But here is a quiz: name the most important protein for constructing your unique size and shape? Have you ever heard of such a thing? The answer is tubulin and microfilaments, proteins that get almost no attention despite being perhaps the most important proteins in defining the fundamentals of our experience. Alpha tubulin and beta tubulin combine to construct tiny tubes called "microtubules." Microtubules generate the cytoskeleton of cells but they are also interstitial (meaning they are in between cells) at super tiny nano sizes and play an unheralded role in stacking cells in an orderly fashion.

Anaerobic fungi are known to produce little fibers called mycelial threads. These can grow inside the human body and when in abundance (called mycelium) will cause all kinds of terrible havoc. Mycelium threads are akin to microtubules and the havoc they cause such as keloid scarring, torqued joints, and malformed tissues are the byproduct of these pathological microtubules going haywire. One reason fungus is such a fundamental problem in the body is that it generates its own microtubules which then become integrated into the latticework of our own bodies. They are not identified as foreign by our immune system.

This means that one reason why fungus is a factor in arthritis is because it alters our microtubule latticework. Fungi are not the only generators of microtubules and microfilaments, which is why this topic has been separated from the topic on fungus above. All cells use microtubules as cytoskeletons which means microtubule and microfilament issues can be propagated by other infectious processes as well.

You can think of microfilaments as being solid fibers and microtubules as being super tiny tubes. Both can get broken, bent, form knots, stunt, unwind (ie. by mercury), and/or grow to excess. If this happens at joints, this is a structural factor in the formation of arthritis – one that won't go away simply by killing off the causative infection.

Once they are there, they are there.

The best way to address microtubule injuries such as these is to follow the advice in this book early enough in your life that you are minimizing how much fungus and other pathogens grow in your body. Alas, this is not an option for most people. If you already have arthritis, you should assume your microtubules and microfilaments are already in pathological states where you are most symptomatic.

One way to help the body heal from "pathological" microtubule and microfilaments is to engage in the natural revival processes that come with intermittent fasting. Intermittent fasting, eating only within an 8 hour window every day (and fasting the other 16 hours) activates natural cleansing processes in the body that have been attributed with feeling more vibrant and more youthful. One reason for this is that glucose deficits on a cellular level cause cells to activate genes that are otherwise not turned "on" that play a role in making your cells and tissues more efficient. Cells have natural functions of microtubule and microfilament resizing and reshaping that are activated, which will help your system identify and clear unhealthy cyteskeleton structures. I recommend intermittent fasting 2 to 4 weeks every quarter especially if you have any symptoms of arthritis.

Calcitonin, Parathyroid Hormones, And Excessive Vitamin D

Our bones are constructed out of calcium and there are mechanisms in the body to pull calcium out of the bones for important biological process that most of the time work great but sometimes go awry. The parathyroid generates hormones that, along with calcitonin, and vitamin D all play a role in calcium regulation at the bones. At appropriate levels, everything retains its order and while calcium might be lost from the bones to fuel other bodily processes, there is no major bone loss. Sometimes these hormones become excessive, however, and this can cause rapid bone loss (in the case of calcitonin, the wrong shape – its isomer – can be the major antagonist). While infections in the parathyroid gland (where parathyroid hormones are secreted) and in the thyroid gland (where calcitonin is secreted) can factor into these imbalances, the more common pathway for problems in bone calcium regulation stem from pathogens that directly produce these molecules as pathogen toxins. Algae and moss, when they infect the body, flood the body with too much parathyroid hormone and calcitonin isomers, whereas overgrowth of mites causes excessive vitamin D and parathyroid hormones as well. I do not yet know what kills off algae and moss effectively, but follow the Anaerobic Pathogen Protocol for now – not because these are anaerobes but because a high oxygen environment likely kills them. And use the Anti-Parasite Protocol for the mites. If you have an osteopenia/osteoporosis diagnosis, I strongly encourage you to assume that these hormonal imbalances are a major contributing factor.

Overall Recommendations

If you suffer from any issues presented in this chapter, you should be on an once a day daily multivitamin that has all the vitamins and minerals the human body needs. For mites and pinworm, you will need a solid 3 months of daily multivitamins to restore the minerals these organisms depleted from your system. But there is no reason not to simply add these supplements as part of your daily habits. While everyone knows you need calcium for your bones, I believe it is fair to say from the conversation about 21-deoxycortisol, the bones need a lot more fundamental building blocks than you may know. Don't just focus on calcium or you miss a whole heck of a lot. Instead, a full daily vitamin is a very good idea – especially if you generally eat the Standard American Diet that is deficient in vitamins and minerals.

Key Takeaways:

- Pathogens attack in colonies which is why they are hard to clear and cause recurrent infections

- Pathogens and their toxins cause arthritis and soften bones but the array of organisms that do this are more varied than you might expect and the strategies necessary to clear these must be robust. Quarterly clearing of fungus and anaerobic pathogens is highly recommended
- Take a daily multivitamin as a basic strategy to remineralize your bones
- Every 4 months, you should eat within an 8 hour span and not eat for a 16 hour span for a 2 to 4 week period to help your cells and tissues renew themselves and clear malfunctioning microtubules and microfilaments

The Joints: Canaries In The Coal Mine

I am 18 years old in high school. I am wearing my brand new ocean blue varsity jacket I earned by playing four years of varsity sports. I am a preppy, handsome young guy, beaming with confidence. High self-esteem is an energy in high school that attracts. I feel appreciated, desired, self-actualized. My grades are fantastic as I have two pursuits: sports and academics as a scholar athlete. I feel whole and complete.

Fast forward four months after graduation, now settling into college. I am sick every weekend. Stress streams through my blood like fuel to a combustion engine. The light is gone as I stare into the blackest of black. I feel burdened and morose. Except for a few fireflies, I feel alone, abandoned, bedraggled, rejected, and unappreciated by contemporaries and professors.

I have experienced an epic, pschyo-social whiplash. I am beside myself, depressed, and speeding towards the bottom floor of self-esteem as if in a rocketship in the gravity of a black hole. Bloody hell. What happened?

That same question: "what happened?" is something we might also wonder in relation to our bodies as they age. There are moments where one day things feel fine and the next, a symptom has popped up that thereafter feels relentless. Often, this demonstrates in our joints. Perhaps you are like me, when you think of aging, you think of older people rubbing their aching, liver-spotted hands as a symbol or totem. There is a basic logic to this: the joints are the canary in the coal mines – locations of regular wear and tear. It should come as no surprise that the areas with maximal movement will be the first ones to express changes in the body.

I am 49 years old, playing tennis against a gentleman who is better than me but whom I want to impress. He runs me ragged side to side. I try to be light on my feet in order to get on top of the ball before it passes me. He hits to my left and I thrust my right foot hard on the ground in order to gain enough purchase as to make a mad dash. But unlike the thousands of other times I have done this very same thing, this time there is an immediate spike of pain and I instantly know I have a problem.

For the next eight months, pain moves all around my heel, never sticking to one location long. As a clinician who deals with other peoples' discomforts every single day hour after hour, I am totally flummoxed. Finally, the pain fixates to a specific joint, the calcaneus cuboid joint and the thick fog of confusion clears. I have torn a ligament in this joint. My work can do many wonderful things but it cannot reinsert strands of ligament that have sharply pulled out of bones. Fortunately, I can walk on it fine and I subsequently walk thousands of miles and play hundreds of hours more of tennis over the ensuing years.

It is today. I am 51, and I have a chronic low grade pain in my right calcaneus cuboid joint of the foot that mostly isn't there but sometimes is. I have a chronic pain for which a surgery is just as problematic as no surgery. I am a terrific clinician, but aging has won this set. I can foresee this pain will be a companion for however much longer I walk and sometimes hobble on this earth.

Most problems are fixable and some are not. Most joint issues have a solution and some don't. Up until I injured my foot, I have fixed every joint issue and injury I have experienced in sports and there have been many. I am not surprised, however, that the chronic issue that has lingered is one at a joint. When you think about machines breaking down, they don't tend to break in the middle of the fuselage; they break down where there is movement and motion – sometimes electrons in motion but mostly where gears communicate.

Our joints are made up of bones into which softer fibers attach. If the bones change shape or these fibers become too loose or too tight, problems arise. Joints also tend to have cushion tissues such as cartilage and bursa, tendons that overlap them, muscles attached to those tendons, and a myriad array of nerves, blood vessels, and lymphatic vessels. There are 350 joints in the human body. How many of these are bothering you right now? Probably very few if any at all. Which is to say, even though there is so much going on in these centers of flexibility and mobility, things are going right almost all of the time. But sometimes they don't.

From a Western perspective, joint problems unrelated to sports injuries are normal facets of the aging process. These are expected and most people will suffer from some auto-immune issues leading to arthritis or bone degeneration reflective of osteoporosis and, smack your hands together, "that's that." I have yet to find a gerontologist or even a primary care physician pull the five alarm emergency cord evacuating the fire houses over a patient's new thumb joint pain. There are just so many thumb joint pains that statistically speaking why wouldn't you expect this patient or the next to have one?

My perspective is very different and it has to do with a fundamental belief that aging is often a byproduct of actual solvable problems. While I do not disagree that as we age we are more vulnerable due to a host of reasons (ie. poorer circulation, changes in blood pressure and blood sugar, and emotional viscissitudes as dear friends and family members suffer, get diagnosis, and sometimes pass away), I do not think even a single joint pain is a "just aging" issue. Often, it is a symptom of a deeper process that needs to be addressed not just to stop this ache but to keep new ones from manifesting via a deepening or progressing crisis.

My patients know that when they bring me new problems they never had before, I am almost assuredly going to talk about this type of infectious organism or that one attacking them. I am a broken record. And I am a broken record because this is exactly what I perceive – most changes in the body are predicated on a problem that is entirely within the realm of our ability to treat. Even my right cuboid calcaneus bone could have a surgery if I didn't think the rehab would be worse than the problem. There are interventions available. But most of the interventions in my play book relate to infectious disease rather than a scalpel.

Why did I suffer in college when I felt peak a few months earlier in high school? Infectious disease. Why did I experience a sudden change in the state of my cuboid bone that allowed ligament tissue to pull free? Yes, I still see this is fundamentally a consequence of infectious disease. As I have already said in this book, we live in a microbial soup and 99.99% of the time, our bodies handle this with aplomb. But every once in a while, something gets through our massive, impressive defenses. When that happens, invariably we will express symptoms. Sometimes those symptoms are acute infection symptoms with congestion or a fever, but often they are much more subtle symptoms that appear completely unrelated to infections – such as a new thumb pain.

The greater question that needs to be asked but rarely is: "why do I have a new thumb pain and does this causative factor threaten my body in other ways?" Because let's face it, if you have a new thumb pain, more often than not it is a harbinger of an even newer thumb pain on the opposite hand shortly thereafter. We tend to say, "well, I was just overcompensating" to explain this newer pain following the original pain. The reality, however, is that pathogens love symmetry. If they attack one side of the body, if left without an appropriate response, they will attack the other side as well, in due time. Why they like symmetry I honestly could not tell you. But it is a fact. If you are seeing symmetry in problems you are facing, don't think "over-compensating" think "infectious pathogens."

The fundamental rule that I am sharing with you is this: any new symptom requires a vigorous response. The "it's just aging" explanation is potentially submission to a greater problem with longer term ramifications. The sooner you respond to something new, the faster you will rectify it and the more likely you will avoid a cascade of new issues and deepening of older ones. What I am advocating is this: fight "aging." That totem in my mind of a liver spotted hand being massaged because it hurts – that is not destiny. The "it's just aging" retort is frankly a cop-out and needs to be rejected. Fight aging. Sometimes it will win a set but sometimes you will win a set, a set you otherwise might have just given up on when you were down the first few games. Sorry, I am drifting too far into my tennis analogies.

I have had many joint pains in my life and I feel fairly young at 51. I have had fingers feeling as if they were changing their orientation relative to each other and toes seemingly starting to torque in wrong directions. I have had injuries up and down my body from sports but I have also had random pains that have come on out of nowhere. If tissue didn't literally pull out of bone, your chance of reversing the process is very high especially if you fight aging the moment it presents itself.

Does this mean the average eighty year old with aches and pains widespread will be able to reverse them all after years of simply addressing them symptomatically with Ibuprofen or Acetaminophen? It doesn't necessarily mean that. But does it mean you have a chance of "reverse aging" as I call it, seeing improvements, reducing intensity of discomforts, and reducing the frequency of discomforts, while also keeping new ones from developing into chronic ones? Yes, I believe so. As I said earlier in the book, it would have been best to have read this book in your mid thirties because you can fight each new discomfort as it arises at the moment it presents. But you start where you start.

So far I have talked about arthritis and bone softening/degeneration and obviously these are issues that will directly impact the joints. Later in the book, I will discuss the torquing of fingers and toes out of position. There are other issues that afflict the joints such as bursitis, edema, and pains of all sorts whether stemming from blood vessels, nerves, soft tissues, or more. In Chinese medicine, there are energetic causes for these problems. But I learned early in my career that if I did not become an expert in infectious disease, I would solve very few of my patients' woes. Which is to re-affirm, most issues have an infectious root.

The toolset for addressing this has already been addressed to a great degree because these tend to be the same types of factors repeating. In the ensuing chapters, if there are problems generated by different types of factors, I will express different strategies. But I think this is a very good, basic strategy:

- As a rule, any new pain needs to be countered that same week and preferably even within the first three days that it manifests. Delay allows pathogens to deepen and they are most vulnerable at the onset of an infection. Even if the pain is the result of a clear and obvious physical trauma, fungal pathogens immediately start to grow in the traumatized tissue, slowing the healing process.
- First, assume the problem is fungal in nature and treat with anti-

fungal strategies. You may feel worse the first 48 hours after starting these strategies but that is not a reason to stop but a reason to continue, as at the very least it is confirming the issue. If after three days of these interventions the pain is neither worse nor better from the intervention, continue these interventions for two weeks but next

- Assume the problem is bacterial in nature and use tools that kill bacteria. The problem should not worsen more than 24 hours after an intervention. If after three days of interventions you see no improvement, then continue these interventions for two weeks but next
- Assume the problem is anaerobic in nature and use tools that kill anaerobic pathogens. Apply for three days. If you do not see improvement within three days, continue these interventions for two weeks but next
- Go on 1000mg of cinnamon a day in capsule form, which will improve circulation in your body. If after a week of cinnamon there is no change, schedule an appointment with a healthcare professional that works on these types of pains and start PT or other therapies.
- If the pains continue, talk to your physician about taking an over-the-counter pinworm medicine and follow the anti-mite regiment as these might be pulling minerals from your bones.
- Throughout this period, take a daily, full multi-vitamin supplement to restore electrolytes and minerals. If the problem is from insufficient minerals in the bones leading to chipping or degeneration, it can take up to 3 months for the issue to resolve. If you have a mite or pinworm issue, the multi-vitamins won't actually start to work until you have killed these organisms that are robbing you of what you need.

There are exceptions to this rule and these have to do with Western medical emergencies. If you are worried you are having a heart attack, stroke, aneurysm, or cellulitis (a skin infection that also comes with a fever), go to the emergency room right away. This protocol I have just described is by no means an alternative to Western medical emergency care for true medical emergencies. Rather, this is a protocol for new pains or any new symptoms in the body (ie. sudden changes in blood pressure or blood sugar or mood) with the goal of stopping them in their tracks early.

If you have old pains in the body, you can use this same protocol I just described to see if it moves the dial, but the window needs to be widened. Your interventions should be a month long rather than 2 weeks. You should give two solid weeks to each stage to assess if there are any changes before moving on to the next step. But don't ever capitulate to aging. Aging will eventually beat us all, but if you fight it, you can slow its victory down significantly.

Even with all of these interventions and more, sometimes a pain is a pain for life. I make no promises. But never assume that is the case. Fight the good fight. I still fight my cuboid calcaneus pain periodically and, notably, it is not a constant pain and I have worn the tread down of many shoes since it started. It is a pain I can walk on and play sports on every day precisely because I have not submitted to it. I will never stop fighting it because I fundamentally believe in the body's ability to adapt if you give it what it needs.

Does this mean you need to stop symptomatic care – taking NSAIDs, using heat or ice on the problem, stretching, or more? Absolutely not. Keep up the symptomatic care if you need it. I will say, however, that Chinese medicine is not a fan of icing pains. From a biological perspective, your blood contains anti-inflammatory molecules that help to reduce pain. Icing a tissue reduces circulation to it and this means fewer of these anti-inflammatory molecules getting to where they can help. If you find icing helps, then alternate icing with heating. If you ice alone, the reduction in circulation can persist and even become a new chronic problem in the affected area. But alternating heat and cold will protect the area from this kind of issue by dilating those blood vessels with the heat.

Key Takeaways:

- Joint pain should never be viewed as "just aging" but instead as problems with actual solutions – and most relate to types of infections

- Vigilance is required and strong interventions are recommended when new pains arise. Fight aging and start within the first 3 days of a new pain

The Teeth

It is 1984. I have secreted away three baby teeth from the tooth fairy (whom I know to be my mom). I am a pure scientist at 12 years old. I wonder what will happen to my teeth if I put one in Coke, one in Sprite, and one in root beer. Within days the ones in Coke and root beer have tremendously discolored. In short time, they disgust me so much as a tweenaged aficionado of sugary beverages, I can't take the experiment anymore. The teeth have rotted disgustingly, I have to call the experiment off and throw those teeth in the garbage. On the one hand, this result was exactly what I expected. But on the other hand, I was hoping for teeth resilient to their environment – in other words a miracle.

Let's just start off with a frank fact that I have previously covered – as a species, we eat way too much sugar and sugar is poison. Many of us, myself included as a coffee drinker, coat our teeths with it daily. Sugar is fuel to infections and it is astonishing that brushing our teeth is enough to protect them so substantially from instantly withering away.

It is 1977. I am five years old. We have just moved into a new home. My elder sisters are best friends and want nothing to do with the baby brother in the family. My best friend at this moment in time is my Big Wheel. I spend what feels like hours riding and then pulling the hand break, skidding in every direction. It is me and my big red plastic friend. The wind in my hair is pure delight.

We have just returned from a family vacation and I am stretching my legs after being cooped up in the car for hours, five year old energy bursting through my skin ready to explode.

My sister Biffy and I are bickering. I have no memory over what. She grabs one of my handle bars. I have no idea what compelled me to do it, but my next act is an act that has lived in infamy in my family system. I straight up bit her hand. I could have used words. I could have even shouted my discontent. No. Instead, I turn animalistic. Fortunately, I didn't break skin, but still, it was my fangs on her skin and it hurt like hell. We laugh about it now, but if you have ever played with a teething puppy you know even a small bite is nothing to joke about.

When it comes to caring for dogs (note to the reader: in my early years, ostracized by my sisters, I was convinced I was a dog, kin to Corkie our black labrador retriever, and not a human), I believe as go the teeth, so goes the dog. The teeth for a dog are critical infrastructure. For humans, this may also be true but dentistry has come a long way, with many interventions that can forestall doom. Fillings, root canals, clearing abscesses, dentures, and implants allow us to not be as vulnerable as canines. Cavities may reflect poor dietary choices and poor self-care. Root canals and abscesses reflect infections getting deeper. Chips in teeth can reflect poor mineralization and again may reflect pinworm or mites as a causative factor. But where things grow most alarming is the loss of bone material that can lead to loose teeth, lost teeth, and even the need for bone grafts in order to set implants. Though alarming, this is also shockingly common. So common, in fact, no one blinks about it.

If something is going on with the teeth, you should wonder if the same phenomenon is a factor in aging elsewhere. One theory for Alzheimer's is that this stems from periodontal disease that continues into the brain. There are many aches and pains as far down as the shoulders and as far up as migraines that can relate to root canal infections spreading through the lymphatic system. These are not my contributions to medicine, but known factors – what happens to the teeth may reflect larger issues. Of course, you should treat any infection in the mouth vigorously. If you have periodontal disease, you should make all necessary changes to get this under control.

Yet it is the bones I once again return to. Degeneration in the mouth is a harbinger of degeneration elsewhere. Dentistry is not taught in medical school: it is its own category of medicine. As is common in Western medicine, categories often do not intercommunicate. A dentist is not likely to be emailing your gerontologist that you have bone degeneration in the mouth and that this should flag, say, a fresh dexascan (bone density test). As a consequence, we, the consumers of this medicine, don't find ourselves even thinking there is a healthcare bridge to gap. If we learn we need a bone graft in one area of the body, rarely does this raise any concern about other areas of the body. But it should. We all have to be the interdisciplinary thinkers because Western practitioners don't provide this service. When a problem shows up in one area of the body, only we will be the ones who might wonder if this crosses into other domains of medicine. And only we will be the advocates to encourage other categories of medicine to poke around.

The breakdown of teeth material and jaw bones are usually slow. But there are times when it can be shockingly swift. If you have ever been a care taker of a dog or cat, you may have noticed one day the teeth seemed fine but the next day, there is substantial unexpected rot. This rot is facilitated by pathogens I associate with Clostridium Perfringens, that same factor that causes gangrene that I already mentioned. Once again, it does this by removing the proper allotropic shapes of 21-deoxycortisol and replaces them with chelated isomers of this molecule (the mirror image bonded to a metal), which causes softening. So much replacement happens in such a quick period of time, the teeth quickly melt away and a dark color can be seen in the teeth, the rot, that is the infection.

These same pathogens can do the same things internally and invisibly. You can see it in people who do not take care of their teeth, the iconic image of a meth addict. The dark brown in the teeth is the Clostridium Perfringens. The lack of brushing quickly allows the pathogen to flourish and spread to multiple teeth in short order. It is gangrene of the teeth. Before long, the teeth are mostly melted. I assume the reader of this book is not a meth or heroin addict and is taking sufficient care of your teeth at least with daily brushing if not twice a day, which I think is ideal. The teeth are usually not where the pathogens can grow in most people due to rubbing its colonies off the teeth vigorously. Instead, if there is an opportunity, it is usually at the jaw bones and what I call "teeth to teeth" joints. We tend to not think of the teeth as bones that are jointed together because we tend to not think of our teeth in motion. The reality is that each time we bite the gums absorb pounds and pounds of mechanical force produced by our jaw contracture and distributes this across these teeth joints causing invisible micro-movements. The means the teeth are actually joints and, as I have said before, the joints are the canary in the coal mine. These joints can suffer wear and tear and this can present opportunities for inflammation and infection. I am not a dentist and don't purport to be one. However, in my experience, abscesses are usually infections in these joints. I consider these red flags, especially for anaerobic pathogens such as Clostridium Perfringens. Any wear and tear of teeth and jaw bones needs to be treated locally but considered a threat of generalized disease. Any issue with the mouth and teeth needs to be considered a global threat requiring a global response, following the protocol that I spelled out in the last chapter about addressing new symptoms promptly.

While on the topic of teeth, please forgive a short aside that draws upon a highly contentious issue in our modern society. I am not a huge advocate for most vaccines as a practitioner of alternative medicine. That said, I do believe that vaccines work and that a majority of humans tolerate them well at all ages. I take issue that we give our children too many too quickly, in my opinion – and way too many before the immune system is mature enough to make maximal use of them (the immune system matures at 5 years old). We often hand them out like candy, sometimes giving people of all ages multiple vaccinations at a time. I am not a fan of this.

But I <u>am</u> a fan of a few vaccines specifically. I don't want to see polio return. I think Measles, Mumps, and Rubella are highly contagious and highly problematic. But mostly, I want to advocate for people as they age to get their regular Tetanus shot. I find people become lax as they grow older and tend to forget this one in the rigors of their regular self-care. Yet, in every single cut with metal without exception, I find Clostridium Tetani associated pathogen growing in the wound.

One place this will show up in my unvaccinated patients is in tension in the mouth and jaws. Those who do not get this vaccine are more prone to neurological disorders as they age as well. But I add this point here in this chapter on teeth to point out that if you suffer from jaw tightness and have not received a Tetanus shot within the last 5 to

10 years, I strongly encourage you to get yours as I feel this one really matters.

I know these opinions likely won't make me many friends and I may be left alone to play with my Big Wheel all alone once more.

People who prefer to not vaccinate will not be happy that I advocate any vaccine. And people who prefer everyone gets all vaccines according to all recommended schedules will find any resistance to the vaccine industry repulsive. I do believe there is a middle ground. I hope people will eventually coalesce here. We should be able to talk about this as reasonable people and without any biting.

Key Takeaways:

- Teeth are joints (teeth to teeth) and therefore are also included as "canaries in the coal mine" as to the health of the bones
- An anaerobic pathogen, Clostridium Perfringins, is a major factor in the more serious teeth syndromes
- Tetanus, known for causing "lock jaw," can be a cause of jaw stiffness and facial nerve problems for people who do not receive their regular Tetanus vaccine, one of the few vaccines I feel are absolutely essential for aging in comfort

The Brain

By all accounts, grandpa Stanley was quite a ladies' man. Not just abundant in youthful vigor, he was charming and dapper. It is 1982, I am ten years old. The grandpa Stanley I know has never had vigor, never had charm, and was never dapper. He was a man who despite having had a Parkinson's-like syndrome called Super Nuclear Palsy as long as I can remember, preferred to eat frogs legs at nice restaurants with a high probability of asphyxiating on his food to the horror of my parents who worried every time he would choke his last. Stanley walked in a snail-paced shuffle and said almost nothing. A few times, I saw him say a phrase or two several times in a row and lastly more loudly with anger to get a point out for public discussion, but mostly he was a mind trapped in a body. He would drive in the front passenger seat and push every button on the grill as about the extent of the joy he emanated.

I always felt awkward with Stanley whether I was ten or twenty-two, the year he passed. I loved him but I did not feel any grandpa-grandchild warmth. Our relationship consisted of me playing several rounds of pinochle and a few more of gin rummy with him in mostly silence, on the railing overlooking a Florida pond. He was a mind trapped in a body but how much mind was in there was anyone's guess.

We all want to keep our mental faculties as we age. That is a given. In many ways, life is the mind and for it to reduce in any capacity we suspect means to reduce in life's abundance. That is, of course, a bit of hogwash in that we do reduce in capacity as we age and yet life's abundance can remain strong. We can forget words or even increasingly forget why we entered a room or two or three, or even feel startled that a skill we once had now is unexpectedly forgotten. These things happen and yet we can travel and enjoy the world's beauty, eat great food, hang with friends, and continue dreaming up future delights even though we are no longer cognitively youthful.

No, the bigger issue is not the regular cognitive decline that is a small part of the indiginities that come with the blessing of more cycles around the sun. It is the more extreme forms of decline that we all truly fear, where we lose a chunk of self. Alzheimer's and Parkinson's are perhaps tops on many people's fears. But there are also factors people don't speak as much about, such as losing one's vision or hearing to the point of no longer being able to engage the mind.

I have worked with elderly patients with Alzheimer's and Parkinson's and I have not reversed these conditions with my work. What I tell patients when they come in is that in my experience, I can slow down progression to a crawl but the progression continues. Perhaps, that will one day change with just the right "ah ha" moments of discovery. But at the mid point of my career all I can do is wrestle major cognitive decline with some bad ass skills but I cannot defeat it.

Nonetheless, I have discovered a few interesting tidbits about these diseases. The first, of course, is that there is no one path to Rome. It appears that there are multiple ways one can march into cognitive decline. Here is a non-exhaustive list of some such causes:

- Serious physical traumas including radiation therapy to the brain and brain surgery
- Enduring mold exposures
- Major circulatory declines (often precipitated by pathogens)
- Stomach organ cell migration into the head (often precipitated by pathogens)
- Pathogens that inflame the brain
- Pathogens that reduce testosterone
- Pathogens that interfere with dopamine production

Again, you can see where I am going with this: infectious organisms are major factors in what the Western world regularly points to as genetic diseases. Which brings me to an aside about genetics.
In my work, I rarely focus on genes. I do this because I feel that we are in the medieval ages in our understanding of how genes actually work. We know, for instance, that genes are not always on even if we have them – they must be activated. One can be asymptomatic for decades of life only to have a gene activate that is then associated with a disease. Rarely, do we talk about infectious organisms as triggers for genetic

diseases suddenly manifesting, but I believe this is the reason why what is latent doesn't just stay latent but become active and perhaps persistent in some people and not others. I say "perhaps persistent" because I also do not believe genes once activated must stay activated. You very well may go from latent to active to latent once more if you clear a causative factor for gene activation. If pathogens and their toxins are those activating factors, then I posit that clearing pathogens and their toxins are the key to turning off problems that develop over time rather than ones one happens to be born with. This may be easier said than done.

The problem with infections initiating genetic diseases is that absolutely all of us have chronic infections we do not know about quietly meddling in our cellular affairs. This means that we have organisms in our bodies whose colonies grow over time as we age, deepening any problem that they set into motion, making it harder and harder for any such genetic situation to reverse – because it is much harder over time as pathogens entrench themselves to clear these causative factors. We also have limited anatomy that often degrades faster from genetic or infectious causes than we can naturally restore it. If a pathogen, its toxins, or genes activated by pathogens result in the loss of anatomical tissues that we need (such as the white matter of our brains) if enough damage is done, it is often a one way street. Which is why I believe I can often slow down progression of cognitive and neurological diseases once they are entrenched enough to be diagnosed as a problem, but cannot (yet) reverse their direction. In the future, perhaps we will have ways to regrow anatomy we have lost and reverse the damage to pre-symptomatic levels. That day is sadly not now.

If you are a reader of this book and wonder if I will make bold promises of reversing advancing neurological or cognitive issues, I am not making those promises. Do I think you can slow an advancing issue down from a rocketship to a snail's pace? I have had that experience in my clinical practice, so yes, I think that is possible in many cases. In my mind, that is still a very important victory.

I will go through the list of possible factors that can cause cognitive decline I mentioned earlier, but before I do so, I absolutely must say there is one huge factor for your brain's health: your care for your physical health. And there are two major factors for your physical health: the daily movement of your body and the food you use to fuel it. Daily exercise is critical to a healthy brain because circulating oxygenated blood is necessary to feed every cell in every corner of the cerebrum with the essential ingredients for their moment-to-moment survival. Exercise overcomes limitations in your circulation (ie. plaque build up or sub-clinical anemia, by way of example) and pushes blood to where it is needed. Study after study has proven that being less sedentary and also being more physically active protects against mental decline. The more you sit, the more you lie down, and the fewer miles you walk, run, swim, rollerskate, or paddle, the fewer cognitive years you will get in your current body. Unless you have a back up body in storage, this is a problem. Not everyone likes to exercise alone, so exercise with buddies. Not everyone wants to exercise with buddies, so find great podcasts or videos to listen to or watch. But get it done. It is absolutely and irrefutably essential.

I spoke earlier about the importance of weight bearing exercises but here the true power of cardiovascular exercise shines. You want to make your heart beat faster and push the blood around to every capillary in the brain. The guidance is constantly changing whether 4000 daily steps is ideal or 10000. My recommendation is simple: if you have body that can only move 4000 steps, move 4000. If you have a body that can move 10000 steps, move 10000. But don't do less than 4000 steps a day. There is also no need to run more than half marathons (I believe more than this puts a huge strain on the physique) if your body is capable of that. Bottom line: make sure to move; but listen to your body. I believe 7000 to 10000 steps a day is ideal, but if your body says 4000 is max, then 4000 is max for you.

Eating healthy is also key for a great brain. This is not rocket science. It's obvious and yet it also can be hard to unpack all of the messages in our society about what is good and what is not good. Over decades of analysis, the Mediterranean diet continues to prove helpful as an overall healthy diet – introducing healthy fats, low meat consumption, and high vegetables to one's dinner plate. As the documentary name says: "Forks Over Knives." Forks Over Knives is a good general motto, though lean meats are fine. In this era, the Keto diet has been widely adopted and while you might expect me to have a strong opinion about it after years of treating patients who have followed it, I actually don't. If you like keto and you feel healthy when eating that way, great. However, red meat is hard on the planet from a climate perspective and there are enough known carcinogenic and diabetic relationships with high consumption of red meat, that I personally think this form of meat should be a rarer input in one's diet, with lighter meats being preferable.

That said, focusing on meat is all backwards in my mind. While it does provide fat and protein, I see it as offering no essential value in protecting the brain. Fats and proteins can come from beans and nuts, just the same. Instead of focusing on protein sources which you absolutely need to consume daily, I believe the key to a healthy brain is found in fruits and vegetables along with healthy plant-based fats. Fat is good in many ways as it protects the brain. Omega 3 fatty acids and fish oils have been known for decades as hugely important in protecting cognitive function. With vegetables comes bioflavanoids, anti-oxidants, vitamins, minerals, color, and flavor. Eat enough of all of this scrumptious delight with just the right spices (yay, more plants!) and the protein is just a secondary addition, an after thought. "Forks over knives" (from a documentary of the same name) is just a phrase about "vegetables over meats" as to what you should focus on to fill your plate. I agree with this and there is plenty of science to back this up.

If you are one of those people who have this trance around "I don't like vegetables" then all I can do is shrug. Your life; your rules… up until a point. The anatomy and physiology of your body has its own rules that don't necessarily follow your emotional relationship with food. You can choose a shorter life with more misery and not eat vegetables because that is a choice you can literally make. But I advocate instead that you simply see the cornucopia of veggie options abundant all around the world as your challenge – search like Magellan for what you like. Because probably you just were born in the wrong family or the wrong typography for your palate – introduced to the wrong vegetables for your taste buds. The world has so much more to offer you and we live in a day and age when we can often import foods from every corner of the globe. Vegetable delights from elsewhere in the world might just spark a renaissance for your palate. Seek and you shall find; and your body will thank you for it.

There is also the belief in child rearing that you should

introduce a child to the same food 15 times before you can say it is unpalatable. 15 times can be in 15 different preparations. I hate brussel sprouts, I thought. But then I tried them char grilled and now I like char grilled brussel sprouts which is one more brussel sprout than I liked before. Yes, you might hate soggy canned broccoli. But have you smothered it in olive oil and baked in until its leaves turned brown and crisp? It's like candy. Which is to say, don't give up on vegetables. They are literally trying to save your brain from your last five years wondering how soap works.

You may have noticed I have not yet spoken about carbohydrates and the reason for this is that we have really fucked up carbs in the modern era. Brown rice vs. white rice. Brown sugar vs white sugar. Unprocessed carbs vs processed carbs with added preservatives and excitotoxins. How can you know what is the right kind of carbohydrate when we have so many to choose from; and how can you know how much to eat when these are all sugars waiting for the liver to decide their fate: energy right now or fat forever. Modern food science has literally tricked the tongue into being insatiable (I encourage you to read about glutamic acid, maltodextrin, and dextrin). My guidance here is to go native and focus as much as possible on consuming carbohydrates as close to their natural form as possible. Brown fats. Brown sugars. Yams and potatoes over processed french fries. Eat as many carbohydrates in their natural fibers as possible as these fibers are not just good in filling out the stool in a healthy way, they protect you from absorbing as much sugar inherent in the food while still allowing those sugars to sweeten what you eat.

As I have said, I am no saint. I eat processed carbohydrates. I prefer white sugar in my coffee over monk fruit. Our family has a rule that works for our temperature zone – if it is over 90 degrees, we splurge on ice cream. But I am also thoughtful about my consumption of carbohydrates each and every time I eat them, which I think is the bare minimum anyone should expect of themselves. Know what you are putting in your mouth and think about whether it is the right thing that you need *today*. Know that the least native your carbs are (with the fewest fibers still attached or the more preservatives and excitotoxins added) and the more you eat these, the more diseases are associated with these choices. And then live with the risks inherent thereof according to the pleasures you need to get through the day *today* and also, very importantly, *every day*. No one needs dessert every single day. Sorry. If you have that habit, it is just a habit, and not good for your *every day*. I would encourage desserts as a once a week treat. And keep in mind that one very real scientifically studied test of mortality risk is how often you have french fries within any given week. Fried foods are usually not cooked in healthy fats and are often full of yeasts (the yeast part is not from scientific study but from my own clinical experience). The more you eat fried anything, the more pathogens you add to your body. As you know, that is not so great for you.

If you want to max out the number of potential days you have with a brain firing on all pistons, you have to factor in these two inputs: exercise and diet. While I am going to speak to a whole lot of other factors within your control based on my work, you have to know that nothing is more important than these two keys to your success, which is why I have belabored the topic again, even though I broached a facet of it earlier in this book. Literally, it cannot be over-stated (though this will be the last I speak about it here). An ounce of prevention is worth a pound of cure has definitely proven true. These are universally available preventative factors.

Serious Physical Traumas

The brain is a tissue and you have a skull to be armor around it along with the meninges to be shock absorbers – and yet still it can be damaged. There are multiple vectors of physical trauma that include blunt trauma such as a severe or multiple concussions, infections, introduction of hydrochloric acid by way of migrating stomach cells (I will talk about this more at a later point), radiation therapy for cancer treatment, and surgeries.

The larger the trauma to the brain, the more inflammation, swelling, and edema. The more the space gets filled with fluid or blood that does not need to be there, the less space for the brain material. Cognitive decline is often noted. People with concussions see this right away, though most fully recover. People with concussions often cannot read or focus. It can feel as if they suddenly put a 100 year old's brain inside their heads even if they are fifteen. The same phenomenon occurs with any sizable impingement on the brain matter.

Whenever a tissue becomes inflamed, any pathogens going through circulation will get caught in that inflammation like a fly getting caught in a spider's web. Once those pathogens land in the traumatized tissue, they will colonize it, which becomes a major resistance to fully healing. Fungal pathogens love to attack traumatized tissue and when they do, you have no idea they are present except via a slower than expected healing process. It takes decades before their colonies are large enough to create clear and obvious symptoms.

After any trauma to the brain, follow the anti-fungal protocols outlined in this book. Also, follow the anti-anaerobic pathogen protocols because scar tissue will also form in trauamatized tissue. Scar tissue contains dead cells that are just the right kind of low oxygen environments in which anaerobic pathogens thrive.

Enduring Mold Exposures

I cannot understate how terribly bad it is for you to live in a moldy environment. This is terrible news for most people because most people live in moldy environments where it rains regularly and spores seed the air at every downpore. I have a special 6th sense for mold as I am very sensitive to it. My wife and I looked at 19 homes before we landed on one that did not have a mold issue, in Rochester, NY. It did have a water-intrusion issue that had to be remediated, but no mold, thankfully. Still, we could have made an offer on 19 homes and ended up living with pernicious molds floating in our everyday air. Most people see mold on the windows, smell a musty smell, visibly see mold in the grout and simply live with this exposure because for all intents and purposes, it seems innocuous. However, there are **no** innocuous molds, there are only ones better at infecting with stealth.

If you live in a moldy house, you should suspect that any chronic health condition you suffer from is from the mold in the house. Period. It might not be, but for 99% of the people out there, it is. I have spoken of the long term impacts of molds on the bones but to get to the bones, molds move through a lot of tissues from the airway or gut to circulation to every place you ever physically trauamatized in your body, and eventually to the bone. Or it can start at the nailbeds from a moldy bathtub or shower and move into circulation through that vector.

It is impossible to live in a house with zero mold. But it is very possible to remediate the molds you can perceive visually and by smell and in doing so significantly reduce your exposure.

One very important intervention is to always use a HEPA-grade furnace and air-conditioning filter. Most people opt for the cheapest air filter on the market, whereas the more expensive ones that remove 99.99% of the mold spores in the air are actually part of your medical prevention expenses and worth every penny. If you have a cheap one, change it today. Most people have molds in the basement and the air intake in the basement will distribute these spores to every room in the house. A furnace filter that clears these spores is far cheaper than working on a frozen shoulder or a foot pain from the bone spurs the molds can sometimes generate, or pulmonary visits for the asthma they can cause. In fact, the array of syndromes caused by mold are so many and so widespread across the body, I can't even begin to list them without creating the impression that these problems are *limited* and not actually your issue when the reality is that if you live in a moldy environment, any health issue you have now or that you developed years or decades ago might relate to it. That is a huge statement, but after more than two decades in my field, I stand by it.

If you have a mold exposure in your home, you should *not* stay constantly on the anti-fungal protocols in this book but should repeat them every month or two. They will lose their power if you over use them. It is better to use them periodically to keep them potent and helpful. Applying 80% bleach solution directly on the molds will kill them. This is highly recommended if you see the mold and can directly address it. Some people will be best served to hire companies to apply expensive mold remediation to their homes. It is unfortunate, but mold affects everyone in the house at every age and needs to go.

Major Circulatory Declines

Alzheimer's is thought to likely be a circulatory disease. It makes sense that if tissues do not get the oxygen they need in order to survive, they don't survive, resulting in the classic brain shrinking found with this disorder. When it comes to senility disorders, I feel there are many paths to Rome but it certainly makes sense to me that abundant blood vessel plaque can be an issue. Pathogens that generate teeth plaque are also associated with Alzheimer's, suggesting any plaque is a problem, likely because it impairs blood flow so significantly.

Cinnamon is actually one of the warmest herbs in the Chinese medical pharmacopiae. We say it goes so deep, it heats the blood vessels. We use it to improve circulation and to clear what we call "Excess Cold" that has invaded the interior. Studies have shown that it also clears up excess triglycerides, cholesterol, and plaque. Some people run very hot by nature and if that is you, cinnamon should not be used as a supplement. For everyone else, two weeks every quarter on 1 gram of cinnamon a day is a good idea to help clear the blood vessel walls. If you have known cholesterol or plaque issues or have a family history of senility disorders, 1 gram a day for a month is a good idea every quarter.

Stomach Organ Cell Migration

The next one is a bit of a weird one. If you are familiar with Endometriosis, a process by which uterine cells migrate to other locations of the body but survive in the new location and continue to be active according to the menstrual cycle, then you will better understand this concept. The stomach cells do the same exact thing. If an infection attacks the top of the stomach organ near the superior stomach sphincter (known as the Cardiac Sphincter), stomach cells can get dislodged and then move with any reflux upward into locations that you might not suspect. There is a Western medical disorder known as Barrett's Esophagus, where this phenomenon affects the bottom of the esophagus leading to symptoms of reflex and GERD. However, enough reflux and these cells can make it to the eyes, sinuses, lungs, and into the inside skull. Wherever they land, they will continue to produce stomach acid, a very strong acid known as hydrochloric acid (pH 1).

In the eyes, this can cause chronic eye dryness. But inside the skull, it can damage cerebrum tissue. Unfortunately, outside of my variety of energy medicine, I do not have a solution for you as to how to clear these migrating stomach organ cells in the wrong locations. You can, however, periodically neutralize the acid by introducing molecules that are of a higher pH, known as bases. I recommend ⅛ teaspoon of baking soda in ¼ cup of water three times a day for 4 days once every two months if you have any history of chronic reflux. If you were to apply this therapy every day, it would not be a good idea as it might contribute to kidney stone formation, which is why I recommend periodic interventions instead. If you have a history of kidney stones, you might want to skip this preventative. Please note that I am saying "baking soda" like drinking a soda and not baking powder, which is not the same thing despite such a similar name.

Pathogens That Inflame The Brain

In my work, I have found many many many many many pathogens are able to attack the brain. We like to think that the Blood Brain Barrier is a firmament like the Great Wall of China but it has no magic properties that can keep pathogens that are determined enough or chronic enough from eventually working their way to the brain. That said, I do not associate most pathogens with the formation of amyloid plaques and Tau proteins, which are specifically associated with senility syndromes. Of those that do, there are two that stick out as main culprits in brain inflammation: Bornavirus and Toxoplasma Gondii. Both of these organisms always co-infect together as a colony. If you have one, you have the other, plain and simple. Toxoplasma Gondii is a single cellular protozoa and Bornavirus is a virus. Together, they increase albumin, which increases transforming growth factor, which causes brain inflammation. It is now thought that amyloid plaque and Tau proteins are actually part of the brain's immune response and a reaction to brain inflammation and not necessarily the cause of Alzheimer's. Bornavirus and Toxoplasma release toxins that cause depression and are my number one "go-to" pathogens to check when my patients suffer from depression no matter if it started yesterday or has been ongoing for multiple decades. These pathogens also increase anxiety and can boost anger as well. If you are seeing memory issues showing up along with a host of negative emotions such as these, then you should consider it likely that these pathogens are part of the picture. Unfortunately, these are not easy pathogens to clear using at-home tools as one organism is a parasite requiring anti-parasitic herbs and the other is a virus, which can be hard to address with supplements. However, if you suspect these as factors, pulse two weeks on and two weeks off supplements that work on parasites and viruses such as black walnut and colloidal silver and see if you feel your memory and mood improves over the course of six months. There may be homeopathic "Nosodes" available for these pathogens, I am not sure as it isn't my methodology. If so, you might consider these. And, if you have really jumped into the Wild West of self-care, you can use Rife Machines to try to kill these buggers.

Another pathogen that I associate with amyloid plaque is Propionibacterium Acnes, the same pathogen that causes most cysts to form in the body. This is a bacterial pathogen. If you have history of cysts or vertebral disc herniations, then suspect this pathogen if you are having memory issues. Pulse colloidal silver two weeks on and two weeks off for six months.

Fungus can also infect and inflame the brain. However, if you are following the protocols I have mentioned in the Fungus chapter, this will help the brain as well.

Pathogens That Reduce Testosterone

People with low testosterone don't just spontaneously develop this issue. There is a causative factor and from my perspective it is always infectious. A huge array of pathogens can be responsible for this, unfortunately. Some pathogens will reduce testosterone while others will build up what are called "isomers" which are mirror image molecules that the body recognizes as if they are testosterone molecules but cannot do anything functional with them, resulting in a net loss of testosterone. Both situations can be helped by going on Western medical testosterone patches, if tests show low "T."

One tell tale sign of low testosterone is a drop in vocal strength. This should be a red alarm if you or a loved one experiences this.

In terms of supplemental self care, you can think of testosterone as made by other hormones and boost those hormones. Progesterone converts to androstenedione and then testosterone. DHEA also along a separate pathway converts into testosterone. I recommend trying DHEA supplementation to see if this helps, unless you also have a need for progesterone supplementation according to Western testing. DHEA is hugely important for brain function and memory, which is why I suggest this method first. I recommend going on a DHEA supplement for 1 month and then assessing if it helped. If it did, repeat this once a quarter.

Of course, this does not address the underlying causative factors, which are pathogenic in nature. Every branch of infectious disease has pathogens within it that mess with hormones and so there is no great singular approach. My main focus in this situations is fungus as fungal pathogens tend to put a huge emphasis on screwing around with people's major hormones such as reproductive hormones, androgens, and steroids. This means following the anti-fungal protocols will likely help. But they also might not, and if the T continues to be low, then next try colloidal silver pulsing it every two weeks for 6 months, as this will help to reduce viral and bacterial pathogens. If low T persists, than follow anti-parasitic strategies. Follow this order as it is the most likely pathway. That said, if you have any history of Lyme disease, follow all of these strategies simultaneously instead as any such pathway is equally likely.

Pathogens That Interfere With Dopamine Production

Dopamine is considered a factor in Parkinson's. Parkinson's tends to end with senility. Which is to say, what if senility disorders have the same root as Parkinson's, but this root is immediately attacking the brain instead of slowly meandering its way to the brain as it does with Parkinson's? In my work with patients with dopamine disorders, I have identified several pathogens that produce isomers (those mirror image molecules) of enzymes necessary to construct dopamine. This appears to be a bigger, more common issue than organisms producing isomers of dopamine itself. There are actually a huge array of pathogens that produce these isomers of dopamine but I have not found that these associate with Parkinson's and Alzheimer's. Once these are gone and the isomers are cleared, my patients continue to be low in dopamine and the disorders continue. Instead, this wrong-shaped enzyme appears to be a much more critical factor.

There are three pathogens that produce it that I am aware of as of the writing of this first edition of this book: Desulfovibrio, Aspergillis, and Alternaria. Two of these are fungal in nature and our anti-fungal protocols will help you clear them. One is a bacteria that specifically reduces sulfate, a sulphur salt. Sulphur is one of the warmest molecules in our human experience and an essential atom for every cell of the body.

If there are signs of Parkinson's or neurological tremors, first follow the anti-fungal protocols. If that does not seem to move the dial. Add colloidal silver pulsing on two weeks and then off two weeks for 6 months to help reduce any potential Desulfovibrio in the body. Also, consider epsom salt baths three times a week (or if you live near hotsprings, hotspring baths) for six months to see if boosting sulfur improves mind and body.

Miscellaneous

Low testosterone results in less motivation, less vital force, and less activity. As the saying goes, if you don't use it, you lose it. Maybe I just made up the saying. Nevertheless, if you don't use your brain, you will lose it. This is one reason why studies show the number one best thing that you can do to protect your brain is to learn a new language. Why? Language involves so many centers of the brain – memory, visualization, sound, planning, and more.

Key Takeaways:

- Unfortunately, there are many pathways for brain dysfunction. The good news is that anti-fungal protocols can help most people
- If anti-fungal protocols don't make a dent, pulse colloidal silver two weeks on and two weeks off for a total of 6 months to clear any bacterial factors
- If these approaches also don't move the dial, go on anti-parasitic protocols to reduce any protozoa in the system
- It is best to try to differentiate which of the above categories you might fit into, as there some unique suggestions (ie. sulfur baths or DHEA supplements) depending on the circumstances

The Eyes

It is 1992. I have befriended many freshmen who are experiencing a Pass/Fail semester at Harvey Mudd College (a semester where there are no grades, they either pass or fail their courses). This means two things: 1. I am hanging out with kids who have never been away from their parents this long. 2. Life is pretty sweet, as there is little pressure this semester – no great weight upon these students to get tons of work done. Notably, I revisit these friends their Senior year after many brutal (graded) semesters and many of them look just plain wrecked. But I am digressing. It is 1992 and a friend has invited me and another friend to his house in San Francisco for Thanksgiving. I joyfully agree to this, especially with the explicit agreement that we stop at Yosemite National Park, a life goal of mine. I am a tremendous fan of Ansel Adams and all semester, I have been full of desire to recreate some of his astonishing photographs at Yosemte.

We enjoy two lovely days pampered by parents who are delighted to have their child back home. Thanksgiving was splendid and our bellies are full. But I am still of one mind about being a cosplay photographer at an apex location. It is time for us to leave in order to make it to Yosemite in time. My friend's feet have suddenly stepped in instant super glue. No doubt he is torn between a lovely pampered life with generous and wonderful parents and going back to living in a dorm that smells of alcohol and vomit and cheesegrate his spirit through the darkest end of the year, the concluding month of the Fall semester. An hour passes and he doesn't budge. Another hour passes; there is no motion out the door. Finally, after a third hour passes, he hits launch velocity and we are on the road.

We drive on the highway for hours from San Francisco to the national park as I watch the sun arc through the sky. The sun hits 50% by the time we are off the highway and 45 degrees by the time we are meandering on switchbacks to the park's entrance. All I want to do is take photographs of this stunning environment and my heart is sinking with the sunlight. Finally, we hit the entrance of the park and the sun is literally at the very tops of the tallest trees. We drive through the first few miles to the visitor center and as we do so, the shadows grow taller and taller until they are taller than the trees casting them and the "golden hour" hits its crescendo.

We exit the car and it is now all shadows. I can't see anything but walls of dark pine trees. There are no mountain peaks visible anywhere. We pee and the dark side of dusk has fully blanketed whatever landscape remains. I can barely make out the shapes of the park offices. I can see nothing that car lights won't illuminate. There is no option to spend the night here as classes start in the morning. I have taken no pictures. I have seen no vistas even though I know they surround me. I am shattered.

We grab a bag of potato chips and some Cokes, get back into the car, and we leave. Maybe we spent 30 minutes at Yosemite total. I saw none of it. And, for what it is worth, thirty two years later, I have never had another opportunity to return.

At 52, I am fortunate that my eyes are doing just fine. But for many people, they know there is a world of visual delights at the ready but like Yosemite's vista after dusk, it is the eyes losing their luster that diminishes the visual experience. For instance, cataracts are extremely common as people age. The eyes also change shape and blurred vision especially when looking at objects up near the face is all but universal. No one wants to hit visual dusk when cornucopias of colors alight the soul. While there are operations that can replace so many parts of the eyes – cornea, lenses, and fix retinal detachments, the reality is that there are also limits that one can reach as one ages that are often undisclosed. For instance, surgeons will balk at additional surgeries if they feel the eyes have hit their interventionist limits. Also, as people reach the goldenest of their golden years, they tend to become much less mobile, much more home bound, and need what can feel like insurmountable support from others in order to go to doctor's visits, which can at times serve as a major barrier for regular eye care. I have had my share of patients who could no longer read books or watch television due to these challenges. For avid book readers, this is far worse than visiting Yosemite at dusk in its heart wrenching agony of the soul.

I am not promising that this book will protect you from all possible eye issues, as the eyes are a very vulnerable organ. They are the only organs that we have partially inside and partially outside our bodies that also need to move around to do their jobs. They must not lose their shape as their shape is vital to their structural integrity and function. Meanwhile, these organs are assaulted daily by viruses, bacteria, and fungi, they are vulnerable to the sun's UV rays, with sunlight being necessary to enter them to do their job, and they are exposed to a world that isn't gentle where even a little flying gnat or the tiniest of hairs can scratch and irritate them. It is a marvel that they weather so much with so few complaints, actually. But it is not a wonder that by people's sixth decade and beyond, the wear and tear tends to build up enough as to be symptomatic and problematic.

There are five main issues to consider in regards to eye health:

1. Visual strength
2. Shape of the facial bones making up the eye orbit
3. Eye pressure, which can impact the optic nerve at the retinal junctions
4. Clarity of the eye lenses
5. Macular swelling and inflammation

Visual Strength

Obviously, the goal of the eyes is to determine shapes and objects and their relative distance to the observer. This is true across all species. Those with the strongest eyes (ie. birds of prey) rely on their stellar visual acuity for their survival and can see a mouse from near a mile up in the sky. I have never been so lucky. I have had an astigmatism my whole life but only in one eye, which means I rarely see a perfectly sharp visual field. But I have strong enough vision that I do not wear glasses, do not need readers (yet), and pass my eye tests just fine (so far). Human eyes don't need to be perfect, it turns out. We just need to be able to make sure we are not hit by cars and know the speed limits, know when our bus is coming, identify the products we want to buy, and turn fast enough so that the bozo from high school we are trying to avoid doesn't see us. Still, we do want to see as maximally well as possible as a basic human desire. Blurred vision is one of the most common complaints in my clinic. No one wants to see diminishment in one's visual power. We might not be catching mice from a mile away, but we still want to maximally enjoy the visual delights around us.

Chinese medicine has worked on visual acuity for literally millenia. We say that the main issue with visual strength is how much "Liver Blood" we have. Liver Blood is not blood from a Western perspective. Yet, when one is anemic, visual acuity is likely to suffer, which means there is a relationship between Liver Blood and circulating blood. It took me most of my clinical career to figure out what that relationship was. As I see it now, "Blood" from a Chinese medical perspective often relates to electrolytes, necessary ingredients for life unknown to the Sages of ancient Chinese medicine. Yet they figured it out their own way – identifying foods and herbs that restored Liver Blood and, in doing so, restored stronger vision among a myriad of other benefits it bestowed across the mind, body, and spirit. Specifically, I have come to believe that Liver Blood and magnesium are the same thing, especially super tiny sizes of magnesium.

The eyes are lazy organs. They will work only as hard as they need to. From my perspective, this is because they rely on muscles which are Earth Qi in an organ that is Wood Qi. Wood Qi controls Earth Qi, which means it is prone to make Earth Qi weaker. Ergo, visual acuity is prone to weaken because muscles internal and external to eyes are energetically vulnerable. Yet, they can be restrengthened fairly easily through one of two mechanisms: 1. Increasing magnesium or 2. Exercising them. There are many known eye exercises and facts are facts, these work AMAZINGLY well. The problem is that eye doctors don't teach them and people are not disciplined in applying them. You would be astonished by how quickly your eye strength can improve with the slightest amount of eye muscle strengthening exercises. But to make a habit of this is challenging. As I have been giving you a calendar for self-care, let's add eye exercises for one week every quarter as an additional strategy. You can find online videos and books about which eye exercises to do so I won't explain them exept in the most basic manner: move your eyes up and down across your visual field from right to left. Next, move then right to left across your visual field from the top of the visual field to the bottom. Move them in spirals starting in one direction from tight spirals to wide spirals then move them in spirals in the opposite direction. And move them diagonally several times in each direction. I chuckle because this is so easy, it is flummoxing. Eye exercises are like kegels – there is a part of the brain designed to make you forget to do them no matter how hard you try to remember.

As to magnesium supplementation, there are many forms of magnesium. Some of these help with gut motility and are also useful for constipation such as magnesium oxide and others are good for the brain and sleep such as magnesium L-threonate. If you don't have constipation as an issue, use the L-threonate. Follow the directions on the bottle and continue to supplement until the eye strength returns to recent better strength. This will only get you back to where you were most recently, it won't make your eyesight stronger. For that, do the eye exercises. Lastly, I will add, that the best magnesium for the body are only offered at sizes of scale found in food, generated by living creatures. Eating foods high in magnesium regularly is even better than supplementation. Examples of high magnesium foods include: dark chocolate, tofu, whole grains, seeds, avocados, certain fish, nuts, and more.

Shape Of The Facial Bones Making Up The Eye Orbit

The body is always in flux, changing in many ways both visible (ie. wrinkles) and invisible (ie. bone density). One invisible change can occur in the bones forming the eye socket. Not even opthalmologists talk about the eye orbit. It is as if the eye exists completely independent of the world of forces around it.

Just as bones in the hips can lose density and this can show up in a Dexascan as a sign of osteopenia or osteoporosis, any bone in the body can lose density and, as we age, most do. This is visible on the face when the soft tissues are no longer held taut by bones that help to fill out their shape and stretch them, leading to extra skin that folds and hangs as a clear arbiter of the aging process. The same process also occurs in the bone eye orbits, which can lead to undo pressures on the eyeball, affecting its shape. It is very likely that this plays a role in the need for readers as one ages, when a person who might have started off myopic (near sighted) over time develops far sightedness and a greater difficulty if not impossibility in reading or perceiving fine details close to the face.

This change in visual field acuity is considered permanent and for all intents and purposes it is. Therefore, it is best to avoid it as long as possible by protecting one's bone density. To this end, you want to make sure your vitamin D levels stay in a healthy range – neither too high or too low. Most people who live in climates that experience three or more months of Winter are prone to vitamin D deficiency and should be on 5000 IU of vitamin D a day between the Autumn equinox to the Spring equinox. It is important to keep tabs on magnesium and calcium levels, especially in women, and even more so if there is a family history of osteoporosis. Supplementation of these may be necessary as well. I recommend bringing a nutritionist into our healthcare team to help you plan a healthy diet that protects your bones.

On top of this, we want to avoid pinworm and mites, as these are factors that deplete minerals from the bones and which will cause sudden acceleration of bone density loss. If you experience negative changes in a Dexascan or bone fracture or any significant injury where you suspect a chip in the bone, you should follow protocols for clearing these forms of parasites. See the chapter on *Bone Softening* for protocols for these.

Once the bones in the eye orbit lose density and close up reading has changed, there is nothing you can do, unfortunately. Therefore, prevention is everything. I would say that you should also look at persisting changes in your visual acuity as a warning about your bones in general.

Eye Pressure

Glaucoma is the condition where the pressure in the eye has increased, which threatens to exert too much pressure on the optic nerve. In my experience, this is an issue of the anterior eyeball chamber and has its roots in infectious processes. I often find pathogens infect the ciliary bodies of the eyes that hold the lens in place, capillaries or blood vessels in the anterior eye chamber, or, very commonly, infect the iris muscles directly.

As is the case for most conditions of the body, there are multiple paths to Rome and I am not asserting the three factors I am about to mention are the only ones. However, it is common for me to find one of these issues in these tiny blood vessels: pregnenolone building up to excess or cholesterol and blood vessel plaque building up here in the eyes. Pregnenolone causes nitric oxide to be released and this leads to chronic dilation of blood vessels/capillaries, leading to a form of swelling that I call "blood cushions," where too much blood occupies the tissue. The impact of cholesterol and blood vessel plaque on the blood traveling through the blood vessels is akin to twisting a hose into a tight loop – sometimes it is closed off and nothing gets through but more often the momentum of the blood exerts a greater pressure. Lastly, the same pathogens that generate cysts in the body can cause hot hormones to build up in the anterior eye chamber leading to edema, a chronic build up of fluid.

There are three varieties of pathogens that tend to be factors in these processes. A fungal pathogen I associate with Stemphylium Vesicarium tends to cause pregnenolone to build up. Bartonella pathogen, a bacterial pathogen that people are often exposed to either from pets or from tick bites, causes cholesterol and blood vessel plaque to accrue. And Propionibacterium Acnes, an anaerobic bacteria that is the most common cause of cyst formation in the body, can be an additional contributor.

It is hard to know which of these is the factor in any person's particular situation in terms of self-diagnosis, but there can be clues. For instance, Stemphylium Vesicarium causes plantar fasciitis and also ADHD, by way of examples of its common negative influence. Signs of one or the other, increases the odds glaucoma is from this factor. High cholesterol, a diagnosis of arteriosclerosis or blood vessel occlusions, pets with this diagnosis, and/or a history of tick bite tends to point towards Bartonella. A history of cysts in the body or vertebral herniations is a good indicator that Propionibacterium Acnes is a factor.

I have listed protocols earlier in the book for fungal, bacterial, and anaerobic factors and I encourage you to follow these. Meanwhile, I do **not** recommend putting anything directly in the eyes (ie. colloidal silver spray) as a way to address glaucoma outside of medicine prescribed by a doctor, as eyes are prone to infection and people tend to trust that their supplements are appropriately preserved when they can in fact be contaminated.

Clarity Of The Eye Lenses

I have spent much of my career trying to figure out cataracts. Even if only in "the beginning stages," I often hear this diagnosis from my aging patients. The eye lens cells are unique in the body in that they are the only cells that I am aware of that fully discharge their cell nuclei in order to be as transparent of a cell as possible to perform their function in passing light to the retina. Retinal cells are one of the few cells of the body meant to last one's entire lifespan – but that is a hard ask when our lives can last many decades.

I now believe there are multiple pathways to develop cataracts:

1. New cells are added to fill in for lens cells that died off – but these replacement cells do not discharge their nuclei
2. Cholesterol and plaque build up in the lenses
3. Microtubules and microfilaments that shape cells and tissues have become bent, broken, knotted, or too many have built up in the eye lenses

The eyes are exposed to the sun and the UV light from the sun can damage cells and kill them. It is generally though that this exposure causes cataracts. When eye lens cells die, they need to be replaced like any other cells in other tissues of the body. However, the discharging of the nuclei, which happens in utero, doesn't occur in adulthood, at least not to as an efficient degree. As I said, the nuclei are large and scatter incoming light that we otherwise want to reach the retina unadulterated. The amount of this scattering is determined by the amount of damage the retina has experienced over one's lifetime and the amount of replacement cells that have been added that are still containing their nuclei. Unfortunately, there are no supplements or medical interventions that can resolve this issue. Perhaps some day laser interventions might be possible that can clear these nuclei, but that is not an option today.

Secondly, cholesterol and plaque can build up in between the eye lens cells also from processes related to Bartonella. There is very little vascularity in the lenses that would allow statin medications to clear this cholesterol, which is why these medicines are not used for cataracts.

Microtubules and microfilaments make up the cytoskeleton that shapes a cell. What is less known is that these same structures can exist external to cells in helping to shape a tissue and define its size and density. Microtubules and microfilaments can break, dent, bend, knot, and be excessive, negatively impacting the tissues when they are pathological in this way. This also can be a factor in cataract development.

Here is the bad news. There are no supplements or Western medical interventions that can imoprove any of these situations, which is likely why you do not hear about people saying they used this or that product and it completely cured their cataracts. There is also not much you can do by way of preventative medicine. I certainly don't encourage anyone to live their life in a cave to avoid sun exposure. There are operations for cataract surgeries that tend to go well and, unfortunately, this will be a necessary path for many. If you have the same risk factors for Bartonella as noted earlier, I would utilize the protocols to clear this as the best pathway for preventing at least this one type of cataract from forming.

Oxalates and other crystals can also build up in the eyes. Archaea are a category of infectious organisms that appear to generate enough minerals/crystals in the eye lenses as to scatter light. At present, there are no Western or alternative mechanisms to clear these crystals once they have built up but perhaps one day these crystals might be effectively treated with vibrational therapies that pulverize them safely. Unfortunately, this is not an option today.

Macular Swelling And Edema

Many people receive a diagnosis of Wet or Dry Macular Degeneration and it is often said that the cause of this is unknown. However, if you have read this far, you know my basic thesis is that most problems are driven by infectious disease. Infections can get anywhere in the body and this includes the eye retina just as much as anywhere else in the body.

There are two main causes for edema (chronic swelling) in the eye retina: fungal pathogens and Bacillus Thuringiensis, a common soil anaerobic pathogen. Therefore these respective protocols are necessary. Furthermore, by now in the book you should see how incredibly important prevention is when it comes to clearing fungal pathogens on a regular schedule from your body as they can grow anywhere and lead to edema and dysfunction. My recommendation for any macular issue would be to very aggressively apply the anti-fungal and anti-anaerobic pathogen protocols for two reasons: 1. The eyes are critical infrastructure that you want to protect them as much as possible and 2. The less vascular a tissue (fewer the blood vessels in a tissue) such as in bones or eye retinas, the longer the intervention that is needed to improve the situation. I would therefore recommend that when you apply the protocols to clear fungus and/or anaerobic pathogens from the eye macula, that you go full months at a time, pulsing every other month, rather than one or two weeks every quarter. Pulsing is helpful because any intervention loses its effectiveness if utilized on an endless basis mainly because pathogens adapt to their circumstances very effectively.

Key Takeaways:

1. Add eye exercises to the last week of every quarter, to habituate them
2. The eye orbit can change shape as an early sign of osteopenia. If you need readers, ensure your diet is helping to maintain your bone density
3. Glaucoma is almost always an infectious process and by either bacteria or fungal pathogens
4. There are multiple pathways for cataract development and no Western medical remedy or supplement yet exists to relieve any of them, unfortunately
5. For macular degeneration, aggressively apply the protocols in this book to clear fungal pathogens and bacteria

Hormonal Rabbit Holes

It is 1976. I am four years old. My dad enjoys fishing on Canandaigua Lake. My whole family – two siblings, parents, and myself have rented a small motor boat at the South side of the lake where the lake is quietest and a great spot to fish. I am bored on the boat. I have youthful energy and I am crawling out of my skin needing to express it – not be cooped up in a boat that is no more than 8 feet by 6 feet and where I have to be quiet so I don't scare the fish. Finally, we make it back to shore and I have gas in the tank. I start running. My sisters have bigger legs and are already out in front of me. I am chasing them around a bend towards a small peninsula where they are laughing together. There is a band of grass along this bend and it is a clear shortcut to get to them. I don't hesitate but run right over it. Except it isn't grass at all. It is some kind of grass-like plant rising up from the water. It is thick like a lawn but it is imposter grass. As soon as I am a step in, I am instantly underwater, as it is already deeper in the lake here than I am tall.

My dad scoops me out of the water – frightened, embarrassed, drenched, and shivering. But lesson learned: not everything is as it seems. Beware of imposters.

I am going to make a huge assertion and you are free to judge me by it. I believe I know far more about hormones than any other person on the planet right now. This is not to say I know every variation of a hormone (ie. 11-betahydroxyandrostenedione compared to regular old androstenedione) and it also does not mean I know the enzymes that convert one hormone into another all that well, which I will admit is a huge missing link in my current understanding, as enzymes are hugely important as I have come to see. However, I have spent years getting to know hormones not just as molecules but as emotions, as triggers of specific nerves in the body (what I have dubbed "subtle muscles" or nerve "switches"), and sometimes even their spiritual importance – as in what they attract into one's life's experience when one hormone or another is elevated or insufficient.

By way of example, there is a gland not yet known to Western medicine that is behind the pubic bone and also by a nerve plexus immediately next to the penis and vagina that when filled with androstenedione, 5-androstenedione, and 11-betahydroxyandrostenedione generates libido, builds vaginal fluid, and also increases pleasure at orgasm. Androstenedione relates to lymph drainage and relates emotionally to "height" as in being above the fray (if excessive, even "elitist"). It can increase a sense of pressure (ie. libido is a sense of sexual pressure). The wrong shape of it, called an isomer, causes being bent over physically (not necessarily in a pathological manner) but also increases curiosity. If a metal bonds to the isomer of this hormone, it can cause "failure to thrive." It plays a role in nerve switches at the back of the eye lens that helps with vision. Ivy plants produce it as a toxin. None of what I know is backed by peer reviewed science and you can honestly say I am only making fundamental assertions without evidence. That would be a very fair rebuke. However, my role in society is to heal people and what I vowed as a practitioner when I was just beginning was "to do what works" as a guiding principle. Therefore, I only can convey to you what has worked for me in my experience and you can take it or leave it. But then again, that is effectively the basis of this entire book – the insights of a single practitioner after tens of thousands of patient visits. Take it or leave it, that's your call. Or you can take parts of it and leave parts of it. It doesn't have to be all or none.

I have written an entire book on hormones for my students in which I elaborate fundamentals of my understanding about hundreds of molecules. In this particular book on aging, hormones constitute only a chapter and not a full tome and so I am going to introduce you to some basic theory. If you wish to learn more, you certainly can learn my energy treatment method called Eminus Mirus (EM for short) and you will find my book on hormones called "Hormones {{{Revelatory}}}" at the EM 4 level, which is the highest level of my educational program.

As basic theory, it is essential for you to know the following: there are hormones and then there are molecules that pretend to be hormones and the body uses both of these because both are found in nature. "Hormones" in my parlance are the proper shape of a protein molecule, known as its allotropic shape, that serves a regulatory role in the body – as in it modifies cells, tissues, glands, and organs in specific, repeatable ways. We say there is a proper shape but this is actually a misnomer as any single hormone can actually have multiple functional shapes (this might be a controversial subject to the handful of biologists among us). You have to understand basic organic chemistry to understand the difference between a hormone and imposter molecules called "isomers." Every molecule has a basic orientation along an axis. Think of your own body standing in front of a mirror. You are the real deal but the image opposite you looks like you and yet is also not quite right. It has flipped sides. Your right side in real life presents as the left side of "you" in the mirror. Any birthmarks on your face change sides in the mirror image. The real allotropic shape of a molecule is like you – it, like you, has a specific design along an axis – an axis defined in an up/down and left/right orientation. The imposter molecule is like your mirror image – it looks a heck of a lot like you but it is wrong on the left/right axis. A molecule having a functional unit on its right side and its imposter having the same functional unit in all respects except it is on its left side, is the equivalent of you having a birthmark on your right side but in the mirror it is on the left.

When it comes to hormones, there are actually three basic types of imposters:

1. the mirror image molecule, known as an isomer
2. The correct shape of the molecule but bonded to a metal it should not be bonded to. This is called a chelate
3. The mirror image molecule, the isomer, bonded to a metal. This is called a chelated isomer

A metal bonded to the correct shape of a hormone is an imposter not because it is the wrong shape but because the weight of the metal makes the hormone behave completely differently than the regular shape of the hormone. A chelated isomer behaves completely differently than the isomer would also because of this same added weight. Metals bonded to molecules so tremendously changes the behaviors of these molecules that these are effectively different molecules for all intents and purposes. Take an average Joe and then fill him up with heroin. Joe on heroin acts like a drug addict whereas average Joe acts normal. The behavior is completely different even though fundamentally Joe is still Joe in almost every other respect. When it comes to hormones, behavior is everything. You want your dopamine to act like dopamine, not heroine addicted dopamine (by way of a silly rejoinder). Though these concepts may be new to you, they are not new to nature, which has been conceivably creating all four types (proper shape plus three imposters) of these molecules since the first single cellular organisms started to become more sophisticated in their actions and interactions.

The human body evolved with "nature" having already figured out these concepts billions of years earlier, which is why our bodies actually sometimes utilize isomers, chelates, and isomer chelates to differentiate the wide variety of emotions we feel. Oh, I need to take a step back and describe something very critical: hormones are emotions. Period. You won't find this in any medical text books except perhaps in relating the effects of dopamine on seeking rewards, endorphins making you feel good, and serotonin in relation to uptake inhibitors to treat depression. But *ALL* hormones are emotions. They are the exact same thing. The reason we can differentiate between attention, interest, curiosity, fascination, delight, perturbation, repulsion, and revulsion depends 100% on which specific hormones, isomers, and chelates construct these feelings (and so many more) that define the full spectrum of the human emotional palette. If they are in circulation, we are bound to feel their associated feeling. When a whole lot of hormones are in circulation, we might feel a jumble of emotions.

As I said, you won't find any of this in any Western medical books. You won't find this information anywhere but here, because the complexity of identifying a single hormone's emotional flavor is such a complex and daunting task, it would be very hard to isolate these molecules within thousands of test subjects in scientific studies. This is no ding on Western sciences – it is simply a very very hard thing to study. Also, who is going to fund a study on which hormone creates arrogance and elitism?

Again, this is not a book on hormones – though the subject is truly exciting and mesmerizing – but on the aging process. Therefore, I am going to pull us back to the task and only discuss a handful of hormones and the roles they play in the aging mind and body. We'll go down a few interesting hormonal rabbit holes and leave the rest of the hormonal universe to your imagination (or your future Eminus Mirus studies).

Before we do that, however, I need to have an important aside with you about cholesterol. Cholesterol is the most maligned molecule in our modern age. While it is differentiated as HDL versions as "good" and LDL versions as "bad," nevertheless, my own physician father would love to add statins to our water supply like fluoride to help reduce all of the vascular diseases that are attributed to elevated LDL cholesterol. Most people have never heard how important cholesterol is to the body. Yes, it is a nerve and blood vessel insulator and helps them perform their functions. True. But the real importance of cholesterol is that it is the precursor molecule to some of your favorite hormones – reproductive hormones, natural steroids that reduce inflammation and improve heart performance, motivating hormones, hormones that generate your value system (thinking of you, cortisol), and hormones that keep your tissues from thinning (we're about to talk about this one).

Furthermore, a very specific fungal pathogen called Stemphylium Vesicarium causes high cholesterol by pulling it out of the nerves and blood vessels where it is needed and subsequently throwing it into circulation. When this happens, there is the impression of high cholesterol because cholesterol is only diagnosed as what is floating in the blood, when in reality the cholesterol is low where it is needed – the nerves and blood vessels. People with this condition tend to be very sensitive to statins, because the blood vessels and nerves are unable to heal themselves effectively without adequate reservoirs of cholesterol that the statins remove. While I do not have a good solution for how to remedy this failure to diagnose low cholesterol in nerves and blood vessels when for all intents and purposes a person appears to have high cholesterol in the blood, what I do offer is the anti-fungal protocol and the cinnamon protocols as alternative considerations in the case of high circulating cholesterol. Studies have shown that taking 1 gram of cinnamon daily for a month lowers cholesterol and triglycerides in the blood. It is a good natural statin. But the bigger issue is that a fungal pathogen is the deeper root of many people's high cholesterol issues. Therefore, anyone with high cholesterol should follow the quarterly anti-fungal protocol and see if over time one's cholesterol score improves. I recommend this even if high cholesterol runs in your family or you have genes for high cholesterol.

The reason why I suggest these procedures is that it is absolutely vital to protect, yes protect, your cholesterol and not overly control it precisely because so many important hormones are literally built by modifying the original cholesterol molecule to make them. If you are low in cholesterol including artificially by taking statins, over time you can become low in all reproductive hormones, low in motivation, and thin out your soft tissues, among a litany of potential woes. You won't find doctors taking this stance as they are very very focused on keeping the Standard American Diet from killing their patients via arteriosclerosis, so focused on this (and let's be fair, that's entirely valid as this is the number one killer in the United States) that they won't tell you that cholesterol is as much an ally as it is an enemy, if not more so. Why they don't take on the SAD diet instead is beyond me, but this is where we are.

One last important aside on this overall hormone topic: our bodies are designed with enzymes that are very shape specific. They mainly work with the proper allotropic shapes of hormones. They are mostly inoperable when it comes to isomers, chelates, and isomer chelates. Furthermore, if you don't have an enzyme that fits a hormone, you cannot break it down. It can persist forever. This means that most isomers, chelates, and isomer chelates that build up in the body have no break down mechanism and therefore they have nowhere to go. They simply build up like refuse inside your tissues. I believe the build up of this molecular garbage is a big part of the aging process. But it gets much worse. The body often recognizes isomers, chelates, and isomer chelates as if they are the proper shape of a molecule – which is a very bad thing if you cannot clear the imposters. When this happens, the feedback loops that would normally indicate that the proper shape of a hormone is too low in the body and more needs to be manufactured malfunctions and one becomes chronically low in the usable, functional allotropic shapes. This failure to make hormones sends cells, tissues, glands, and organs into a tailspin that also is a major factor in the syndromes and diseases often attributed to aging, such as chronic muscle weakness, depression, possibly Alzheimer's and Parkinson's, plus so much more.

Since no one in Western sciences yet realizes this problem with imposters, no one is intervening with solutions. Instead, we are stuck exclusively dealing with the symptomatic care of so many issues. That said, it probably would not be all that hard to create molecules that attach to isomers and rid them from the body. The science is there. What is needed is the knowledge that this is a genuine issue and the right biomedical corporation seeing dollar signs as an incentive to act.

Pregnenolone

First there is cholesterol. Add Cholesterol Side Chain Cleavage enzyme et voila: pregnenolone. Pregnenolone is the first in a very long chain of hormones differentiated only by an enzyme or two or three that fill out some of the most important molecules to make the news: testosterone, progesterone, all of the estrogen varieties, cortisol, androgens, and even more natural steroids like cortisone and cortisol. Pregnenolone functions by increasing nitric oxide, a potent blood vessel dilator. This causes capillaries to expand where the pregnenolone is located. It turns out there is an optimal amount of expansion of tissues. If you have too little, tissues thin out and people get the diagnosis of thinning membranes (often incorrectly sold as a natural facet of aging). If you have too much pregnenolone, the problem is one of too much blood in a tissue, which will create what I call "blood cushions" that are a chronic form of swelling in the body, akin to edema but different (edema is made of fluid cushions whereas blood cushions are full of blood). These cushions can show up as unsightly bumps on the surface of the body but imagine what those same bumps can do internally to say the kidney organs, the liver, blood vessels, the spinal cord, and more. Bumps are bad. Blood cushions are a problem.

It turns out that the same annoying Stemphylium Vesicarium fungus is the main culprit in most cases of excess pregnenolone causing blood cushions. It does this by pulling the cholesterol out of position and using enzymes to convert some of it into pregnenolone. It then breaks down the enzymes that convert pregnenolone into other hormones. Like a dam on a river, it forces the body to make pregnenolone in excess. Likely, it does this because it prefers these blood cushions as areas to chronically infect – with easy access to blood and its circulating nutrients.

The most common cause of thinning tissues, a big issue when it comes to aging, is a build up the isomers, chelates, and isomer chelates of pregnenolone. Since no enzymes work with these molecules, the body is tricked into thinking it has pregnenolone when it actually doesn't have enough and so does not make new proper shapes of pregnenolone, resulting in a chronic constriction of capillaries and blood vessels and, subsequently, a chronic thinning of tissues. The good news is that if you experience this, you can take pregnenolone as a supplement. The bad news is that the isomers, chelates, and chelated isomers that have built up don't have a natural or supplement/ pharmaceutical mechanism to be cleared, which will result in the need to ingest pregnenolone on a persisting basis to take over a function the body should otherwise satisfy naturally. In other words, without a mechanism to address the problem, you will have to deal with it symptomatically on an ongoing basis.

Estrogen & Progesterone

The hormones you hear the most about are estrogen and progesterone, the celebrities of the hormonal universe. Yes, they are important. But to think of any one hormone being more important than another when it comes to the hormones generated by cholesterol, that is kind of silly actually – each is critical in living a full, contented life. Nevertheless, you have no doubt heard about the importance of these hormones when it comes to perimenopause and menopause. Of course, they are important in how they change over time, but the story, as often is the case, is more complicated than how it appears on the surface. Women's eggs produce hormones and as the eggs diminish, these particular hormones eventually diminish to the point that the menstrual cycle ends. Women who have oorectomies (removal of the ovaries) experience early onset menopause, confirming this assertion. Often, this is blamed on the reduction of estrogen and progesterone produced by the eggs, though I am of the opinion there is another hormone that controls the overall menstrual process on a macro level (not talking about gonadotropin that controls it on a cyclical basis month to month). It is true that if you put a woman on replacement hormones, this can cause the cycle to return – but this is only because progesterone creates a lining in the functional zone that will once again shed, creating the impression that progesterone is the key to retaining a cycle. I mentioned androstendione earlier. I believe this is produced by the eggs and is the ultimate determiner of whether a women is in her fertile wisdom years or post-fertile wisdom years.

It is extremely important to note that men and women have estrogen and progesterone. Similarly, women have testosterone. There may be relative differences among the genders but in reality there can be women with excessive testosterone and men with excessive estrogen and this is common. In this subchapter, I am talking mainly about women, but all issues that women face in regards to estrogen and progesterone, men face as well just as often. It just is not as evident as the cycle provides a more obvious sign of what is going on internally. People often do not realize there are three basic subsets of estrogen: estriol, estradiol, and estrone. And, among these three subsets, there are multiple variants such as estriol 3 glucuronide or estradiol sulfate, by way of example. Each unique estrogen has a completely different function in the body from the next one. Add to this isomers, chelates, and chelated isomers, and you will find estrogens can go haywire in all kinds of interesting ways. The same is true for progesterones. Estrogens and progesterones move sodium and will engender swelling and water weight where they build up excessively. People with chronically too much estrogen tend to have a pale, puffy, swollen physique with soft tissues and weaker muscles (from being swollen).

These are also “hot hormones” and inasmuch, wherever they build up, edema (chronic swelling) follows. Between pregnenolone, estrogen, and progesterone, you will find 60% of the causes of swellings in the body followed by androstenediol and glucocorticoids making another 20% (the last 20% relates to histamine, in my experience). As you can imagine, when estrogen and progesterone are excessively high, it can be very hard to lose weight especially since so much of this weight is water weight – a facet of the sodium building up from these hormones. Water follows salt wherever it is located in a process known as "osmosis." This means anyone with high estrogen or progesterone resulting in high sodium will retain water. Since the only mechanism in the body to excrete salt is via sweating and people in our modern times tend not to sweat sufficiently while at the same time eat the Standard American Diet which is dangerously high in sodium, salt builds up more and more over time in our bodies leading to the expected phenomenon that people add more weight as they age (attributed to a slowing down of metabolism), which is far from a requirement of aging.

I have two major problems when it comes to estrogen and progesterone and they both relate to a complete lack of knowledge of isomers and chelates. The first is that women are regularly diagnosed with imbalances in these hormones without any differentiation of whether they are high or low in the correct shape of the molecule or one or more of its imposters. The second is that the remedy for most hormonal imbalances with these hormones is bio-identical hormones and yet pharmaceutical companies regularly make products that I have found to be full of isomers, which might look exactly like the correct hormone except it is built along the wrong axis and is, as a consequence, a different hormone altogether (an imposter), serving no satisfactory role in supplementing where there is a deficiency. Which is to say, "Houston, we have a problem." Women are regularly being misdiagnosed as to their hormonal problems and are being offered remedies that aren't actually remedies.

If you are likely to find a physician who knows the height of what there is to know about hormones from a Western medical perspective at the peak of today's knowledge, it would be functional doctors – whom I love. These are the doctors who will test what can be tested and really do their best to get a complete assessment of one's molecular truth. However, they are hampered by a lack of tests and tools that really look at this issue of imposters not just in the blood panels but in the treatment tools available to them. I think any eye rolling by functional doctors right now is partly frustration with me because they know a lot of questions will follow this book and also eye rolling because they know there are limitations they are facing as compassionate practitioners that no one with advanced biochemistry degrees are solving for them. The good news: these can be solved. Modern science can figure all of this out. The bad news: the people in charge today have been clueless to the issue and need to perceive the challenge in order to rise to it.

Suffice it to say, imposters of estrogen and progesterone exist and are a problem for the reasons I have previously stated. There are no enzymes to break them down. They will build up in the body and impact the negative and positive feedback loops that help the body decide what it needs and where it need it and this will result in syndromes and diseases that relate to estrogen and progesterone, in this case. From a Western perspective, there is not much that can be done except to improve their bio-identical hormones to contain as few imposters as possible or to forgo synthetic hormones and focus on hormone replacement via natural products such as yams and vitex berries as these contain proper allotropic shapes of the hormones we need.

It will come as no surprise to you to hear that fungal pathogens are the main culprits in messing with estrogen and progesterone, followed by Bacillus Thuringiensis, a common anaerobic bacteria found in soil. Prevention is the best approach, and following the protocols in thi book in clearing fungus and anaerobic pathogens will protect you as best as possible from any build up of imposter estrogens and progesterones. Please don't get me wrong, every genre of the infectious organism pantheon has the "technology" to create estrogen and progesterone imposters – including parasites, viruses, and other bacteria. You would be hard pressed to address every possible scenario. You can do your best in all respects and then catch Epstein Barr Virus or food borne Hepatitis A and have a skipped cycle or an early cycle due it playing around with progesterone. However, if you clear fungus from your body, you are addressing 90% of the more chronic factors that encourage hormonal imbalances in the body.

This leads me to an aside: if you skip a cycle or have one come weeks early or have a cycle with unexpectedly heavy flow, this is not a cause of concern. It is incredibly common for infectious organisms to mess with the cycle in exactly the manner I just described. Most viruses and bacteria come and go and these blips in the cycle are just blips.

However, a change in the cycle that persists hints at some organism that is chronically infecting. If the anti-fungal and the anti-anaerobic protocols don't address these persisting issues, follow an anti-parasite protocol and see if that makes a difference, by way of suggested treatment strategy.

Okay. That was a lot about women's cycles but I do need to remind you that men and women suffer from imbalances in estrogen and progesterone. Any swellings large or small, weight that is suspected to be water weight, and any heat disorders (remember, these are hot hormones) should be treated as if they stem from estrogen and progesterone imbalances regardless of gender.

Testosterone

Testosterone excess causes tightness. This is different than stiffness. Stiffness you only feel when actually using a joint or tendon but tightness lingers even without use or movement. We tend to think of testosterone from a perspective of impulsivity or libido and to some degree there is a relationship. However, I attribute the bulk of libido to another hormone and while testosterone will make you feel agitated (like you should do something but you don't know what to do) and it can increase impulsive and intrusive thoughts (dihydrotestosterone, a testosterone variant causes this), to the most part, it is an important hot hormone in regulating heart rate (too much and you have tachycardia) and helps you power through tasks that require any amount of persistence.

As men get older, it is common for there to be too little testosterone reulting in a weaker voice, less physical power, and kidney issues. It is my belief that there is a gland in the medial inferior lungs not yet known to Western medicine that has a relationship with the pituitary gland and the parathyroid glands that regulate testosterone. The weakness in the voice is a good indicator that this lung gland that secretes testosterone is having issues. Women also can have issues with low testosterone, but men more often than not appear to suffer the voice weakness. Any sign of a weaker voice, and a blood panel that examines testosterone, parathyroid, and pituitary hormone levels would be a good idea as well.

As noted, tightness relates to imbalances with excess testosterone and more often than not to a build up of the imposter molecules. Many organisms produce these molecules and while my database of pathogens include fungi and anaerobic pathogens plus one or two parasites that I am aware of, more often than not viruses and bacteria play a major role in its production. The list of such pathogens goes on and on from pathogens you have heard of (ie. Streptococcus) to ones you have never heard of (ie. Protomyxzoa Rheumatica). I therefore recommend following the colloidal silver and goldenseal anti-bacterial protocols if tightness is flaring up or a regular, chronic affair.

As noted above, there are many subvarieties of testosterone playing unique roles. Stemphylium Vesicarium, a fungus, increases 11-ketodihydrotestosterone, a potent nerve over-stimulator. I attribute this molecule in the substantia nigra and the corpus collasum as a factor in ADD and ADHD symptomology. People of all ages suffer from this and the older you get the more likely this diagnosis is overlooked for attention or memory issues attributed to old age. As with most fungal pathogens, Stemphylium tends to increase in the body as we age. It is a tree fungus and exposure is highly likely in most people. If attention and memory issues are cropping up, it may be a senility issue but before you draw that conclusion, follow the anti-fungal protocol and see if clearing this pathogen helps improve attention and memory. This is especially true if tightness is part of the picture, and in particular if this is worsening hand-in-hand with memory issues. Stemphylium is the main cause of plantar fasciitis in my experience with the tightness from that also having a testosterone association. If you have any suspicion of this pathogen being in your system, you know what to do! It is a fungus. Crush it.

Stress Hormones

It is a common facet of aging for people to become more sensitive to stress and more anxious over time. Part of this has to do with larger energy cycles of life where one's first 10 years relate to an energy we call Water Qi that has a profound influence on our physical structure. This Water Qi cycle returns in one's 60s when structure once again tends to become a hot topic, but this time not in its developmental processes but where things start to age and, in some cases, break down. Water Qi, when excessive, increases fear, which is one reason why people can experience spikes in anxiety in their 60s (and beyond) that are resonant of spikes of anxiety in one's early years (at times, it might feel like temporary emotional age regression). Changes in physical structure are also highly stressful to the mind and the body, which is a tie that connects these hormones to this aging process.

Stress hormones can accumulate in the thalamic reticular nucleus, the most important part of the brain for sleep, resulting in tossing and turning and lighter sleep, along with early wake ups. Stress hormones also tend to accumulate fat in the abdomen, where it is common for fat to build up more and more as one ages, often attributed to a reduction in one's metabolic rate, and yet so specifically aligned with the area of the body sensitive to "cortisol weight gain." Humans have two essential enzymes that break down stress hormones currently known to science, though others might be added to the list over time. These include MAO and COMT. It is common for people to have at least one broken gene for these enzymes resulting in insufficient break down of stress hormones. People with this situation will swim in stress far longer than those who do not have this issue, also providing ample time for stress hormones to build up more and more in the system. People with this situation tend to avoid stressful situations because it is very uncomfortable to wear this enduring stress for extended periods of time on a psychological level, let alone a physical one.

One thing the elderly are known for is there diminishing life aperture. When they were young, they were zipping all around town, getting into all kinds of fascinating episodes at all times of the day. By contrast, the elderly prefer their "ruts." They prefer the same cycles at the same time of day handled in the same exact way. One reason for this can be attributed to mental processing and executive functioning changes that I will discuss later in this book. Another reason is that they are producing fewer and fewer COMT and MAO enzymes due to a build up of their isomers and chelates. As a result, stress hormones are flowing more extensively in circulation. Any additional stressor will compound this issue.

Furthermore, cortisol in particular will cause connective tissues to overstretch. When you see a person who has lived a very stressful life, their faces are full of wrinkles and they look much older by decades than those blessed with more pleasant circumstances. The reason for this is that cortisol causes overstretching of collagen, elastin, and fibrin – fibers that help to hold one's tissues taut. This overstretching is not just external but also internal which accounts for all manner of stretching and drooping of internal tissues, the source of a thousand problems in the body.

Why is this stretching occurring? Because COMT and MAO proper allotropic shapes are fewer and fewer, resulting in higher and higher cortisol in circulation, leading to more and more tissues stretching.

The number one way to reduce stress hormones from the body is to exercise. It is the backdoor way to break these down because the muscles utilize the stress hormones in their cellular processes. Another way to break down stress hormones is to meditate for at least 10 minutes a day. If you have never meditated, I highly recommend you look up videos on Theravada Buddhist Meditation, as this is a very simple process of focusing on the breath. I also am a gigantic fan of self-hypnosis, a method I feel was early maligned in its history but which is perhaps one of the most profound, under-utilized interventative method ever created.

Obviously, I am a huge advocate for exercising to stay youthful, as indicated earlier in this book. However, there is an alternative to exercise and meditation that you can try and that is supplementation with either Ashwaganda or SAMe. This does not always agree with everyone, but it may serve as a possible workaround for reduced MAO and COMT and therefore for controlling stress as it builds up via the aging process. I am not a fan of supplementing endlessly with this supplement. Instead, one should be self-aware as to when major stressors have occurred: sickness (ie. catching the flu), major injury, surgery, loss of a loved one, marriage conflict, child conflict, and more are moments in time when someone who feels susceptible to swimming in stress would benefit from supplementing with Ashwagandha or SAMe for the duration of the stressful experience (or, in the case of an illness like the flu, waiting until after one recovers from the illness).

It is important to stress that you want cortisol in your system. Cortisol is essential for two vital processes: 1. It gives you a sense of strength in your muscles (without it, your muscles feel weak), 2. It embues value to the things you care about (without it, you don't care about anything and this is a form of depression). Therefore, I want to underline that you absolutely do not want to remove all cortisol from your system, even if it might threaten (when excessive) to cause a wrinkle. Better to have wrinkles but not literally falling over due to muscle weakness. Therefore, you should not go overboard in trying to control cortisol. Yes, it has a dark side, but it also is a critical ingredient to raising the quality of your life. Quite a plot twist.

Thyroid Hormones

Rarely, do we talk about glands being tied together with each other according to their negative and positive feedback loops, but one such important set of glands is a relationship axis between the adrenal glands, the hypothalamus, and the thyroid gland. If one gland goes out of balance, it is very common for the others to follow suit. I just spoke about cortisol going out of control and this is often how conversations about hormones often run – as if they are isolated issues. Yet, we know that glands operate in tandem and that problems in one mean correlating problems in others. Yet, it is very uncommon to hear anyone with hypothyroidism talk about the hypothalamus and anyone with adrenal issues thinking about how the thyroid is relating to this.

As far as I know, and I am no expert in this, hypothalamus hormones are not included in most regular blood tests, though cortisol and thyroid hormones often are. This means, one has two data points for a three data point problem.

It is impossible not to talk about the thyroid and aging, given the tremendously high prevalence of hypothyroidism within the community. It is my experience that hypothyroidism often relates to isomers of T3 building up in the body along with isomers of Thyroid Peroxidase (the proper shape of this molecule is the TPO noted in blood panels). Sometimes pathogen toxins can play a role in hypothyroidism such as thallium, a toxin produced by Botulinum. I should note that most if not all isomers of T3 and Thyroid Peroxidase are pathogen toxins as well. When you feel extremely tired during a bout of the common cold, you are experiencing a bout of temporary hypothyroidism due to the isomers of T3 that Rhinovirus is producing inside of you.

Pathogens are constantly manipulating our thyroid hormones. Some produce hormones that generate hyperthyroidism such as the flu. These hormones generate heat in the body whereas the isomers of T3 generate cold. In fact, I have cured some cases of Reynaud's simply by boosting T3 proper shapes in capillaries of the hands and feet because these warm molecules play a role in blood vessel dilation.

As is the case with medicines for emotional disorders such as depression, it is common for people to suddenly see a major change in their thyroid function despite being on Western medicine, and this is immediately interpreted as the body has changed and a change of dosage or a new medicine is necessary. What is never taken into account is the most recent infection the patient just had. Blood tests are photographs of hormones posing in the blood at that one moment in time. This snapshot provides data but not context. When there is a change in the state of a hormone, the patient's aging process is often blamed or some facet of adaptation, when in reality, it is more likely an indicator of the type of infectious organism the patient's immune system is currently wrestling with or that was only recently conquered. The problem we have is that once again we are dealing with pathogen toxins of a variety that there are no enzymes to break down. The more Rhinovirus a patient experiences in their life, the more isomers of T3 have built up like garbage in the system. The more flu bugs, the more hyperthyroid generating molecules are building up. There are no great interventions at this moment to permanently clear these isomers on an herbal or pharmaceutical level.

I put this example last not only because it is a great prelude to the complexity of glandular interconnectedness (ie. if you have adrenal fatigue, check the thyroid too), but because sadly I do not have a great "go to" tool for you to bring this situation back into balance. What I do have, however, is advice. When the thyroid numbers change, unless there is a compelling reason to do so (ie. extreme, unremitting fatigue), do nothing and test again in a month or two. Take two snapshots instead of one before making changes in dosage or medications. Any change in medication will require your system to adjust to these changes which can cause as much chaos as the problem itself. I advocate being patient and seeing if these isomers continue to sit around like garbage or if your body's liver detoxing, exercise, or other natural processes help to reduce the toxins that were added.

As for self-care, the next best thing I can offer is that you focus on detoxing every time you get sick because the detoxing that happens immediately around an illness strongly determines the amount of garbage left behind to clog your cells and tissues. When you get a cold, flu, stomach bug, a sinus infection, bladder infection, vaginitis, or any kind of infection for which you find yourself feeling significantly hit or needing antiobiotics…focus on detoxing immediately thereafter. I strongly recommend that you take *methylated* B vitamins such as the variety produced by Pure Encapsulated in their B Complex Plus product. B vitamins are unusable when they are ingested. To become usable, a molecular process called "methylation" occurs in which a "methyl group" is added to the vitamin. Only *methylated* B molecules are bioactive and functional. Some B vitamins are essential in constructing glutathione which is essential in detoxing. An enzyme called MTHFR (methylenetetrahydrofolate reductase) is an important part of the methylation process that makes the vitamins usable and therefore capable of creating glutathione. Not everyone makes enough MTHFR enzymes and therefore detoxing becomes a major issue after an illness, prolonging one's state of feeling ill or off. I strongly recommend skipping the methylation process and take already methylated B vitamins in supplement form just in case you might be one of those people struggling to build enough MTHFR enzyme, so that you can build enough glutathione and detox pathogen toxins more efficiently. As I said, this protocol is hugely recommended after any infection so that you can eradicate as many imposter hormones introduced into your body as soon as possible through your own body's natural processes, to help keep them from becoming part of the aging process.

Conclusion

This is just the tip of the iceberg. Our bodies rely on hormones to do so much of the every day and even every moment cellular leg work. I cannot over emphasize their importance. Yet, it is shocking how little is known about them on a therapeutic level. As a result, imposter garbage builds up and feedback loops break down leading to increased suffering across an increased array of bodily systems that sometimes have important correlating relationships with each other. Frankly, it's a real mess, especially if you do nothing. However, I have provided you with some great self-care ideas in this chapter. I hope you find them useful and that they improve the length and quality of your life.

Key Takeaways:

- Pregnenolone controls how thick a tissue is. "Thinning tissues" might benefit from pregnenolone supplementation
- Estrogen and progesterone play a huge role in swelling and in water weight retention. Pharmaceutical companies do not understand that the mirror image shapes of these hormones are actually very problematic and can lead to many side effects – and their products are often inundated with these
- Menstrual cycle issues are likely from fungus if they become chronic
- There are several testosterone variations that each do different things when awry such as tightness, intrusive thoughts, agitation, and ADHD
- Stress hormones cause overstretching and lead to many aging complaints, including joint pains and wrinkling. Regular, daily exercise is the best way to clear these

- When thyroid numbers change in blood tests, at first, do nothing and test again. Very often, this is from recent infections producing isomers of T3 or of TSH
- After an acute infection, focus on detoxing for a couple of weeks by taking already "methylated" B vitamins

Emotions Of Aging

It is 2004. I am a new arrival to Frederick, Maryland. I have signed up to work as an acupuncturist at a group facility run by therapists who have promised me referrals and space in exchange for a sizable cut of my acupuncture practice income plus rent. I am paying rent but not seeing those referrals despite that sizable share they are receiving with each patient visit. The facility is receiving my payments and they write me a check monthly. I am good at marketing and my practice is already growing substantially despite almost no internal referrals. I also am not prepared for the amount of weird ass shit going down among some of the people in that facility. In short order, I am suspecting the manager is a cult leader and the people working are afraid of him or in love with him and in some cases both. I think he is a scuzzbucket. I come to this opinion quickly because I am good at seeing people for what they are.

I up and leave one day on the spot when it is clear that shady things are happening among Mr. Cult and a partner that might impact my professional reputation, plus those referrals are clearly never actually going to come, as, to the most part, it was a bald faced lie. If I stay, I share my income with them for nothing forever. I am owed $4,000 for work I have already done and for which I was not yet paid. I am explicitly told by the Mr. Cult I will never see that money. On that, he was honest. I never do. When asking a partner to intervene, instead I receive a letter telling me I am unethical and a bad person. If you know me, that is a hoot. I am ethical to a fault, if that even can be a thing. But it is the cat calling the kettle black. Narcissists seem to like this strategy, and I am convinced Mr. Cult actually wrote the letter.

I am left with a conundrum – do I sue for what I am due? Do I bring into my life's experience lawyers and courts, stress, and conflict. I have a newborn at home. We need that $4000. Do I suffer for months or years plus lawyer bills and court costs for a $4000 benefit? Some would. But I am a spiritual person and I perceive everything in my life from a spiritual perspective. I see that I am meant to be free and that on *one side is darkness and the other side is light. I see that if I go in the direction of courts, that brings that energy into my field and I might see it again and again in my career. And if I don't, I won't.*

I don't sue. I don't spend my years hollering and waving my fist at people who are twisted. Instead, I trust my choices and my path. I never turn back, and it is the absolute right choice. Let karma have its say. And if karma thought I was unethical and a bad person, it is curious to have rewarded my career with endless wind in my sails and great joy in my heart. I doubt that was the same for that greedy group that from day one didn't keep its word – and I don't care. Once free, one is free.

I share this story because it actually speaks to aging and its emotions in a few spot-on ways. First of all, years are like money, we all wish we could have more, no matter how much we are blessed with. Sometimes, it seems as if aging is a process of robbing us of life for which we somehow feel entitled to simply because we exist. One can dwell on this and lose even more life. One can raise one's fist at the loss of function, loss of degrees of freedom, and also simply dying too young. That useless fist waving is a choice. You could choose it but it won't change a damn thing. Life is not always what we want it to be or what we expected. Sometimes we discover people around us acting unethically or deviously, and we feel there is a personal cost or personal harm from this, and it feels unfair because it is unfair. But fairness is not guaranteed as much as oxygen and water, heartbeats, and aches and pains. That said, one can move towards the light and fairness tends to increase the more yards you gain. The light in this case, is a move towards the positive: appreciation, unconditional love, generosity, and kindness. Fairness is not guaranteed even if one moves in this direction, but chances are higher and certainly you will enjoy a path with substantially more light than you will along a path of shadows.

I will add that often the emotions that come with aging are not choices but forced upon us. When I was put in this lawsuit conundrum, I was stressed out and it was absolutely appropriate for the experience. But we do have choices even when it might seem we don't. We can choose light even when that light seems very dim. As soon as I made my choice not to sue, I was immediately released of the stress and burden. It was only money. My spiritual world was far more important.

In this chapter, I am going to talk about a few common emotions as we age and steps one can take to feel more thrive-y and less sodden by these feelings along the long arc of our aging process.

Sadness & Depression

I believe it is fair to say that sadness and depression are a song whose refrain returns more frequently as we age due to various factors that include: loss of loved ones, a reduction in things to look forward to at the larger levels such as big trips, completion of big projects, sparks of romance and so forth, the load of chronic pathogens building up in the body often containing organisms that secrete sadness hormones, and an increase in isolation that can come with a decrease in mobility.

General Thoughts On Sadness And Aging

From a purely behavioral perspective, while there is nothing we can do in regards to the loss of loved ones as a facet of the human experience, we can intervene on several of the factors that encourage sadness that I just listed. We can make sure to always have a carrot in the future to look forward to by pushing beyond one's comfort zone and planning trips or events. We can force ourselves to be more social and less isolated by joining hobby groups or by participating in/organizing gatherings. And we can attack pathogens in our bodies actively and not accept our physical circumstances as permanent just because they are physical and have been persistent. Much of this book is about this last point as this is not a book on how to find hobbies, how to plan trips, or how to maintain community even as mobility becomes challenged. But I will say one thing about planning for the future – always have your next spark lit for something coming up that you enjoy, even as the last spark is extinguished at completion. If you love theater, have your next tickets purchased by the time your next scheduled play is upon you. If you love travel, already have in mind the seed of the next trip even as you are boarding the plane/train/bus/car for this trip. This is a habit of keeping light in your life. Think of life as a cave and the future as always going deeper. You would never go into a dark cave without a flashlight and extra batteries or a torch that won't easily extinguish.

Five Element Dynamics Of Sadness

Sadness and depression are the same emotions that also generate grief. However, as for grief, these feelings are specificially generated in the lungs, the organ of sadness and grief in Chinese medicine. Metal Qi is the energy of sadness. If you suffer from sadness or grief, you will want to limit Metal Qi in your hobbies, habits, and diet and you will want to increase Fire Qi. Everyone is born with Five Element combinations that create a Constitution and people with strong Metal Qi in their constitutions will also be more predisposed to more intermittent sadness, depression, and grief along with an increased love for Metal Qi lifestyle choices and foods. Unfortunately, these predilections work against your mood.

Metal Qi activities include sports with Metal gear such as racket sports with metal rackets. The exception to this are bikes which are made of Metal but the actual sport of biking is Fire Qi. I have strong Metal Qi in my constitution and I quickly found tennis to be my lifelong sport. Metal Qi foods include earl grey tea, Lapsang Souchong tea, white sugar, spicy foods high in capsaicin, aromatic foods with many spices, lavender flavored foods, and alcohol (every kind of alcohol except beer). If you are experiencing a period of sadness, grief, or depression, I strongly encourage you to reduce these foods. I also encourage you to increase Fire Qi activities and Fire Qi foods. Fire Qi activities are high stimulus, high adrenaline, or constantly changing scenery (which is why biking is actually Fire Qi). Running, dancing, biking, river kayaking, skiing, walking in new locations, and hiking are forms of Fire Qi activities. Fire Qi foods include: black tea, green tea, dark chocolate, coffee, cinnamon, and beer (beer is only suggested if you do not have any unhealthy relationship with alcohol). Beer also encourages yeast issues in the body and so it is a mixed bag, that one.

Sadness has many shades: disappointed, disinclined/inhibited, hesitant, constrained, sad, grief, lacking passion, lacking joy, lacking love, lacking motivation, and so forth. The last four I just mentioned are more often a lack of Fire Qi due to excessive Metal Qi. Another one, lack of connectedness, is a lack of Wood Qi due to excessive Metal Qi. Wood Qi sports have back and forth elements such as swimming laps. Wood Qi foods are sour and include lemon, limes, and cherries. I will add that simply taking a drive is a form of Fire Qi. Simply spending time in a park is a form of Wood Qi. If you are sad, build Wood and Fire Qi and see how that feels. Wood Qi plus Fire Qi makes very strong Fire Qi.

While Metal Qi is the cause of depression, there are always facets of other of the Five Elements that further differentiate it. Depression with inactivity as if life has become frozen is a Water Qi depression. Often one will not necessarily feel depressed as Water Qi and Metal Qi are each low in the actual experience of emotion. But the lack of functional activity is the sign of this kind of depression. People with this kind of depression need Yang energy – they need to to move, they need stimulus, they need action – even if they are sitting down while it is happening around them. People with Water Qi constititions somatocise their feelings which means they tend to have physical symptoms rather than emotions. People who feel fatigue, are frequently injured, or have major enduring pains may be experiencing a Water Qi aspect of depression.

Lack of connection, as I said is a Wood Qi depression. Lack of joy/love/passion is a Fire Qi depression. Both of these as I said are lacking Yang energy as well, as Fire Qi and Wood Qi are the Yang Elements of the Five Elements. They also need action and adventure to help resolve. Travel (especially to new locations) is a healing agent for these types of depression as the action of traveling is Wood Qi and the newness of the experience is Fire Qi. Mostly, resolution comes with sustained habituation of these actions and are unlikely to noticeably change with just one or two Yang adventures. Which is to say, doing something once or twice is not a habit, it is an exception. You need to make a habit that includes Yang and Fire Qi to more easily fend off sadness.

Feeling depression itself as an intense emotion is a sign of an Earth Qi depression, as people with Earth Qi feel their feelings very strongly. Avoiding sugar will be helpful for people with this form of depression.

Hormones of Sadness And Depression

When it comes to hormones and medicines, a major focus in Western medicines has been very off base, from my perspective. Don't get me wrong, many people benefit from medicines they take and the right medicine can turn around depression. But medicines are based on a partial understanding of how hormones work – mainly based on the proper allotropic shapes of hormones such as dopamine and serotonin and also proper allotropic shapes of their receptors (which also can be found in isomer forms, often as a byproduct of infectious disease). However, most sadness, grief, and depression relates to the "wrong" shapes of hormones – isomers, chelates, and isomer chelates. 4-DHEA isomers (mirror image molecules), for instance, generate feelings of disappointment. They are regularly produced by pathogens as toxins and the second these toxins build up sufficiently in the blood, one is suddenly feeling disappointed in others, in oneself, in one's life partner, in one's family members, in life's circumstances, and in work. Once the infection has resolved, the hormones become less problematic, and these emotions mostly recede – but what if the infection is chronic? Then what? There are no medicines that clear 4-DHEA isomers.

Various fungal pathogens increase isomers of serotonin – which creates a frustrated depression. A person with this kind of depression is more likely to be both sad and have sudden negative verbal outbursts or actions. As you know, fungi build up in the body and the kinds we tend to have chronically infect us are ones that often build up these toxins. SSRIs can help with serotonin uptake control but they do nothing to clear the isomers nor do they kill the fungus that is daily producing the emotional toxins.

A Common Pharmaceutical Trap

While this may sound discouraging, there are a few takeaways. The first one is that a sudden change in mood is likely an indicator of an acutely attacking pathogen. What often happens is that when mood worsens, the patient goes to the doctor, the doctor says "your medicine is no longer working" and then what ensues is a painful process of getting off one anti-depressent for another. The new one might have new side effects. When a short-term painful yet better choice is to simply wait one month. Obviously, if one is suicidal, this isn't an option. But barring that, waiting one month allows a viral and/or bacterial infection to work its way through, after which the emotions are likely to return to their previous state and the medicine that "was no longer working" suddenly is back up to snuff again. This saves months of agony of starting a new medicine. Meanwhile, use the protocols in this book to attack all forms of pathogens in the body to speed up the healing process. If the emotions stay worse after a month even after anti-infection protocols and boosting Fire Qi and Wood Qi activities/foods while reducing Metal Qi foods, then yes, it is time to think about pharmaceutical changes – but preferably not until then.

Grief and Its Impact On One's Energy

One last point on grief. Grief is a natural process and it takes time. Unfortunately, it dissipates Qi (energy) and also causes fatigue. It is therefore necessary to keep grief from burdening the system too excessively. The immune system will weaken from the Qi dissipating from the lungs, as the underlying energy of the immune system called Wei Qi will get depleted. I recommend for everyone going through the grieving process to take Astragulus tincture drops for the first three months after a loss to protect the immune system. I also recommend reducing Metal Qi foods and increasing Fire Qi activities and Fire Qi foods to protect your energy. Grief comes in waves and at times may settle for a while during the first year. Any time it sustains for a week or longer, again reduce Metal Qi foods and increase Fire Qi foods and Fire Qi activities. It may be hard to do as a result of the demotivating nature of grief, but it is important that you sustain yourself.

Protecting Fire Qi To Protect One's Mood

The physiology that holds the energy "Fire Qi" includes the heart, pericardium, capillaries, blood vessels, bone marrow, and the small intestine. These tissues need to be full of Fire Qi to protect one from depression. The heart is the organ of love. The pericardium is the organ of faith. The capillaries and small intestines are organs of unconditionality such as unconditional love and unconditional acceptance. Fire Qi itself is increased with laughter, passion, newness, stimulation, and joy. It is each and every aging person's duty to keep these full in one's experience and, when possible, to share them. The easiest way to protect this Fire Qi is to be in community.

Anger & Resentment

Many people experience growing anger and resentment during the aging process, though this is not as assured as grief. For one, we increasingly like what we like and don't like what we don't like – finding ourselves so deep in "grooves" that they can easily become ruts, stopping any further forward momentum and growth. It is easy to become angry when people push you out of your grooves when you might feel you have earned your right to stick to what you like. Resentments also can increase as a consequence of old hurts biting deeper and from feelings of loneliness or abandonment while other younger people continue with life's many enduring demands or as life's compatriots die or are stricken and isolate themselves. Old childhood traumas that never quite healed tend to burn hotter if they haven't been fully processed through therapy or one's own healing journey. And, let's face it, anger and resentment are emotions and we are certainly entitled to them. Often enough, they are justified.

General Thoughts On Anger And Resentment

When you let people live rent free in your mind endlessly, this carries dangers that are often overlooked. For one, anger raises blood pressure. Combined with arteriosclerosis, high blood pressure increases the risk of a heart attack and stroke. Resentment is formed via what we call Energetic Wind, an energy in Chinese medicine we specifically associate with strokes. There is no physiological benefit to holding onto anger and resentment and not much psychological benefit except where it might encourage positive action such as seeking healing of past harms and the remediation of unhealthy relationships. More often, it simply stews like smoldering embers waiting to catch something on fire.

It is interesting to watch animals such as dogs work through anger. You can see anger clearly in their visage and their actions. But then it passes. They shake (known in human healing circles as "discharging"). They lie down. Recoup. And move on. Perhaps, they remain "twice shy" but they don't tend to carry anger into the next moment. Humans clearly have a larger capacity to remember and to hold onto hurts. But we can take from this at least one clear message – moving your body is a great way to discharge negative feelings allowing one to move on. Athletics of any variety are massively positive in purging any acute emotional charge, even if they do not actually provide healing of any underlying interpersonal dynamics.

Arguably, one of the most powerful acts a human can make is to forgive. Easier said than done, that is for sure. Personally, I have adopted the "expiration date" mentality that there is an expiration date to my hurts. Once that date is passed, I consider the individual guilty of generating my wrath having been young and therefore stupid, like a silly, thoughtless child when they engaged in their crimes against me. I then simply choose to forgive them. That is perhaps the most interesting facet of forgiveness, that one can simply select it as an option if so willing. Mind you, I never forget who hurt me and how, I simply never put myself in that same position to be hurt again, and I forgive. I am hardly as quick as a dog when it comes to moving on – my expiration date is 20 years! If I could do it sooner, I would. But carrying anger for longer makes me think I am the silly one. I try to remember that no matter a person's age, they are always emotionally a child. They might be thirty years older than you, but still a simpleton of the heart. Emotions don't evolve and convert from my "youthful anger" to my "wise elderly anger." Anger is just anger. It is a spice of life, but a spice that tastes exactly the same every time it is experienced. It isn't like wine or cheese and improve with age.

Five Element Dynamics Around Anger

Anger is the emotion of the Liver and Gallbladder as it is a Wood Qi emotion. It often comes with shout as the sound of shouting is a Wood Qi sound. Anger can come with rage and violence at its extreme and this only happens when the Yang energy of the Liver rises to the head due to not enough Liver Yin energy to anchor it into the Liver organ.

There are two basic constitutions that tend to experience anger more than other people. The first are people who have Wood Qi in their constitutions. You can spot these people easily because they tend to be loud, often shout (mostly not in anger), easily get hot headed, express anger regularly but mostly at a mild level, and often they are the ones pointing out how they can do things better than how they are currently being done in almost all circumstances. And they probably can.

Wood Qi constitutions simmer more regularly with low level anger. By contrast, people with Metal Qi in their constitutions keep beating and beating and beating on their Liver organs on a Five Element energy level, eventually resulting in not enough Liver Yin anchoring the Liver Yang and then suddenly out of nowhere, perhaps seemingly out of character, a sudden, intense rage is released. Metal Qi people don't simmer with anger regularly and so these outbursts are as suddenly surprising to the Metal Qi person as to those who witness the sudden intense action or release of anger. Where this would feel fine to a Wood Qi person, a Metal Qi person feels uncomfortable and perhaps even embarrassed after an angry outburst.

Hard alcohol is to the most part a Metal Qi food and people who drink are effectively making themselves into Metal Qi people with this same dynamic. Drinking alcohol beats and beats and beats on the liver until the Liver Yin is diminished and sudden rage and anger is released. The number one thing an elderly person who is experiencing increased experiences of anger and/or resentment should do is to stop drinking alcohol. Recent research has determined there is actually no healthy or safe amount of any kind of alcohol, despite earlier studies that had suggested moderate drinking was actually good for you. If it is encouraging increased bouts of anger, it is not just not good for you, it is plain bad for you.

White sugar is also Metal Qi and while its impact is less obvious than alcohol which hits the liver organ as a big blast when one drinks, instead sugar can hit like a blast or build up its impact over time. As people age, they are more likely to develop diabetes, which means higher blood sugar for a sustained period. Getting blood sugar under control is therefore a necessary act for those who are experiencing elevated anger and resentment. Outside of Western medical interventions for this, a very potent way to help restore normal blood sugar is to engage in intermittent fasting, in which one reduces one's eating hours to a specific window of time during the day such as an 8 hour window. For diabetics, this should be done under the supervision of your primary care physician as it may be unhealthy for you to suddenly go from eating throughout the day to suddenly constraining yourself in this manner. However, having purposeful periods of hypoglycemia via this methodology has proven to help improve blood sugar. At first, hypoglycemia periods might increase anger and resentment but only for a short period of time, until the body adapts to these changes, which will overall improve blood sugar and therefore help the liver organ be healthier as well.

Hormones Around Anger

Testosterone has many variants that include ones that increase feeling agitated, generate impatience, increase impulsive thoughts, and instigate sudden unexpected bursts of anger. Androgens are molecules that magnify emotions and high androgens along with high testosterone varieties can tremendously increase anger. You won't be surprised to hear that I find infectious organisms often produce both androgens and testosterone variants (especially isomers, chelates, and isomer chelates) and are often major contributing factors in generating these feelings. Bornavirus and Toxoplasma, which always infect together as a colony, increase sadness, anxiety, and also anger. One is a bacteria and the other is a parasite. Therefore, the protocols for bacteria and parasites should be followed to help bring these under control.

I have come across a few organisms that increase ethanol, drinking alcohol, as a pathogen toxin. These include a fungus called Mucor Racemosus that gets into people via insect bites such as horse fly bites. I have also found a virus that can produce this as well but while the virus is less likely to chronically infect a person, Mucor Racemosus can cause infections that last years. The tell tale sign of this fungus is regularly feeling drunken without drinking anything. Sometimes people experience this as feeling a sense of disequilibrium or clumsiness. If these are showing up, use the fungus killing protocols from the earlier chapters.

There are a few other organisms that directly produce anger via their toxins that would mostly be dealt with following the above suggestions, but there is one exception and that is Herpes viruses. Herpes has many subspecies including Epstein Barr Virus, HHV6, HHV7, Herpes Simplex 1 and 2, and Cytomegalovirus, to name a few. All of these can chronically infect and as a consequence can encourage chronic anger via their toxins. Unfortunately, there are not many great anti-viral supplements that I can recommend to clear Herpes. Given the wide variety of herbs and supplements that have sky rocketed in recent years, I would not be surprised to find that there are products on the market that suggest that they kill off Herpes pathogens specifically, but I have no personal experience with them, so I cannot make any educated recommendations.There are anti-viral medications – but this is a conversation to have with your physician as to whether this is appropriate for you and which is the right medicine for the right problem. Rife machines purport to kill pathogens like Herpes, but can only clear what is actually infecting and not what is dormant and well hidden/disguised.

Pharmaceutical Treatment Of Anger

Anger is not a commonly prescribed diagnosis. Perhaps this is because people who suffer from it tend not to self-disclose their chronic, enduring anger to their physicians – as if it carries some societal stigma. Unless acting out in anti-social ways, enduring anger can be a very invisible issue, especially to health care practitioners who only spend a few minutes with you a year. Likely, medicines for other issues would be used for this such as tranquilizers. There are no "forgiveness medicines" or "trauma-clearing pills." Therapy is often the most prescribed alternative to medicines, and I believe this is actually better than medicine quite often. Nevertheless, I recommend one tries the protocols mentioned in this book to see if this moves the dial on anger and, if any of them do, this does point to an infectious instigator of one's emotional state.

Protecting The Liver To Address Anger

As I said, the liver organ is the key to chronic anger if the issue is not from infectious disease. Increasing Wood Qi foods that are sour in taste (but not excessive in sugar) such as lemon, limes, and cherries may be helpful for Metal Qi constitution people who experience sudden unexpected outbursts of anger. Also, milk thistle can be helpful in restoring balance to the liver regardless of your constitution. Magnesium is an important electrolyte for the liver as it builds what we call "Liver Blood" in Chinese medicine. I would recommend going on regular magnesium L-threonate to further build liver organ Yin.

Fear & Anxiety & Worry

Fear, anxiety, and worry are flavors in this amazing soup of life. Unfortunately, as we age, these are the feelings that constrict our lives more than anything else – often leading to smaller and smaller apertures of activity and movement, smaller and smaller spheres of interest outside of the house, and less physical movement during the course of the day.

There is nothing worse for a person than allowing these apertures of life to shrink – as lack of human-to-human face-to-face contact, lack of utilizing collected life talents (ie. how to navigate the highway system), and lack of the joys and passion of experiencing something different or new will shrink the brain akin to atrophy of a muscle. It will also shrink the generosity of the heart. Life has grooves of what we enjoy and these deepen and deepen and deepen as we get older to the point that the elderly fight against going out of those ruts rather than embrace the adventure of being free of them – which is the superpower of youth. To live longer, you have to live life – which means embracing the discomforts that come with aging and living. Fear is a major factor in people giving up on life. The fear of falling is a huge fear. The fear of traveling with pain is another. I am a person with a phobia and I know how paralyzing fear can be and how terrible and triggering it is. Yet, you should think of fear like a wrestler that you must defeat. You might not win every round, but keep up the fight and you are likely to win enough to make life worth living. We all know people whose lives have collapsed into a bedroom, the kitchen, a bathroom, and the television room – and that's it. Fear brought them to a maximum of 800 square feet of life. This is your enemy.

Five Element Dynamics Around Fear

Fear, anxiety, and worry each worsen as we age. There are actual physiological reasons for this unknown to Western medicine and Western sciences. We live under a sun that is an Earth Qi factory. All day every day we are influenced by what is at the heart of our solar system. I have seen pictures that illustrate that the planet Earth is, for all intents and purposes, literally within the sun itself when you include the sun's winds. This means, the number one truth about living on this planet is that the influence of Earth Qi is ever present.

There are many many wonderful things about the sun and living within its influence. It is one of my happiest parts of life, especially since I live in upstate New York where we have six months of dark gray skies. But there are a few drawbacks. The first one is that Earth Qi plays a huge role in worry, as one of its fundamental building blocks. This doesn't mean living near the equator where you have more days of sunlight and more hours with the sun equates to more worry. It isn't one-for-one like that. It just means that as time progresses in one's life, those building blocks for worry are increasingly likely to generate more worry. Toddlers have all will and no worry, but grandparents? Often quite the opposite.

Second, Earth Qi, according to the rules of the Five Elements, "controls" Water Qi. What this means is that Earth Qi can reduce Water Qi. Water Qi makes up some very important parts of our bodies including our bones, our brains, urinary tracts, reproductive systems, and our legs. Look at each item on this list and you will see that these are locations where most elderly suffer more and more over time. Why? Because the fundamental building blocks of these aspects of our physiology melt over time under the influence of Earth Qi. Are there things you can do about this? Yes! Absolutely. But imagine a clock where you can't stop it, you can only turn back the dials a bit at a time once and a while and you get the idea of how we much we can influence this process.

As Water Qi tissues "melt" under the influence of Earth Qi (and I am using "melt" more figuratively than actually), the Water Qi comprising them moves into circulation and resettles elsewhere where

Water Qi is problematic. Excess Water Qi in the wrong locations feels like anxiety and fear. Which is to say, osteopenia/osteoporosis and anxiety/fear have a very direct relationship according to Chinese medical theory. The bottom line: anxiety, worry, and fear are expected outcomes of being successful at aging. You therefore need to have clear and explicit strategies to counteract this influence because otherwise it can be consuming.

Hormones Around Fear

The hormones that generate fear, anxiety, and worry are each different. There are hormones that generate a feeling of terror and there are hormones that create the physical, somatic effects of terror (ie. shaking/trembling uncontrollably). These may have sounded the same, but they are actually different. There are hormones like neuropeptide Y that generate worry – which I define as repetitive loops of anxiety generating thoughts. Norepinephrine plays a role in worry and isomers of epinephrine play a role in phobia. There are also fight or flight hormones unrelated to these two, regardless of the fact epinephrine and norepinephrine are the most attributed. There is the emotion of agitation, which is created by testosterone, and generates the bouncing off the walls feeling, a sense of needing to do something but not knowing what that "something" is. These are only a few representative examples.

Keep in mind, fear is actually biologically a good emotion as it tends to keep us from doing things that are life-threatening. I don't like heights and probably this is some over-communication of a biological reminder system that getting too close to a cliff's edge might not be so good unless you happen to have goat hooves for feet or feathers. Fear is not a bad thing. It is fundamental and life-protecting. However, when it starts to associate with things that are not life-threatening, such as the fear of walking outside because one once fell and broke a bone, then this is a problem if that fear controls one's choices and behaviors. We don't want to live a life without fear, we just need it to remain appropriate and well-proportioned.

Pharmaceutical Treatment Of Fear

I think it is fair to say that Western medicine does not differentiate anxiety from fear or fear from worry. If you complain to your doctor of worry, it is effectively the same to them as if you complained of anxiety. Even as I write this, you might find yourself scratching your head and wondering if I am a mad man. But the reality is that anxiety, fear, agitation, and worry are all separate issues as reflected in different hormones producing each, as indicated above. Fear is the physiological feeling of fear. It is the panic, rapid heart beats, shaking, shrinking of consciousness, and expression of immediate danger or alarm. Anxiety, by contrast, is a psychological experience. It is does not come with repetitive thinking but a sense of something impending that is wrong with a looming sense of negative potential outcomes. High histamine causes generalized anxiety, for instance, which comes with a generalized sense of something being wrong. Agitation is the need to move because one is so wound up internally. And worry is playing a common playlist of concerning or alarming thoughts that never quite turns off. While this certainly is an exaggeration and my psychiatrist friends will take umbrage, to the most part, each of these is lumped together under the rubric of "anxiety" for which there are many Western medicines. If you want to call me out and say agitation is more likely to be treated with tranquilizers whereas the rest with anti-anxiety medications, I will give you that. But that doesn't get you too far from my thesis.

Unfortunately, what is lost in our modern society is the wide array of self-care interventions that are actually quite impactful for each of these emotions that have been mostly abandoned for pharmaceutical medicines including: binaural beats (music that actuates brain waves that reduce anxiety), self-hypnosis (my personal favorite), glasses that blink in patterns that activate delta brain waves that produce hypnotic and relaxing effects, bio-feedback, aromatherapy, bach flower remedies, and, not to be forgotten, meditation. These are each so very very powerful. I mean really. These are like "super hero powers," powerful. I recommend people who read this book find a self-care tool from this list that works best for them regardless of whether or not you also use

Western medicines. As I said, fear is our enemy combatant; gather your metaphorical weapons people!

Protecting Water Qi Tissues To Fight Fear

Meanwhile, none of these interventions actually deals with the fundamental root cause of fear, anxiety, agitation, and worry. These are all crutches to get through the feelings. My goal is to help you slow down or turn back the "fear clock" as far as possible. To this end, we need to control Earth Qi and boost Water Qi.

First of all, I recommend everyone get regular Western blood tests and review the following: how is your fasting glucose level? Glucose is a form of Earth Qi. If it is high, explore intermittent fasting and dietary changes to help level it. Go off red meat, sugary drinks, white sugar foods, white bread, and daily desserts. Check your vitamin D levels. If it is low, go on vitamin D to protect your bones. Check your creatinine and GFR. If these are out of balance, support your kidney health as the kidneys are the main organs of Water Qi. There are various fruits and vegetables known to help the kidneys. I recommend 6 months on a macrobiotic diet in the case of kidney disease. Check your histamine levels to make sure you are not experiencing anxiety due to new or worsening allergies including to environmental factors and foods.

Water Qi foods are high in calcium and sodium. Make sure you are eating foods that replenish the bones. If you have osteopenia and/or osteoporosis, you want to immediately start weight training as nothing is more protective of the bones than this. Make sure to start off with a personal trainer who can show you how to weight train without causing injury.

Concluding Thoughts On Emotions

Emotions are our guiding rods. We each follow them in a manner that controls our actions. If something makes us happy, we do more of that. If something makes us angry, we tend to avoid it. If something makes us afraid, we often excise it from our life's experience. Emotions are flavors of life and the problem we have when we confine our life's experience to fewer and fewer emotions, is that we have to box ourselves in as well to do so, and furthermore it might make us feel better in that moment to be in our grooves, it does not serve our soul's purpose. If you take only one thing from this book, it is that you should age in a manner that continues to embrace the unknown and the uncomfortable. To do anything else, is to live in a continuously shrinking box that eventually becomes one room, a bathroom, and the tv.

Key Takeaways:

1. Alway have something exciting planned for the future. Keep a bright torch lit as you wander deeper into the cave
2. If your "med stopped working," unless it is a medical emergency (ie. causes suicidal ideations), wait one month – as often this is a sign of an acutely attacking infection working its way through the system
3. Fire Qi increases with laughter, passion, newness, stimulation, and joy. It is each and every aging person's duty to keep these full in one's experience and, when possible, to share them.
4. Forgiveness is a powerful healing method. Strangely enough, one can simply choose to forgive, like choosing lunch off the menu. You simply have to be open and willing
5. People struggling with anger should avoid alcohol and white sugar
6. Chronic anger can be a constitutional factor or from infectious organisms producing anger generating hormones

7. Fear and anxiety are the worst for constricting one's life as one ages and this must be fought against with every fiber of your being
8. Just being on the planet long enough causes fear and worry due to Five Element dynamics that involve the sun and our planet Earth "melting" the Water Qi off of our bones. Water Qi excess is felt as fear and anxiety and Earth Qi excess can be felt as worry
9. Find a tool on this list and make it your fear-killer: binaural beats, meditation, self-hypnosis, bio-feedback, bach flower remedies, aromatherapy, or deep abdominal breathing
10. Fight fear and anxiety by weight training
11. Continue to embrace the unknown and uncomfortable as a guiding mission in your life at every age

Menopause And Other One Way Roads

I am 17 years old. Though I am ranked 3rd in my region in tennis for my age group, I have never won a tennis tournament. The reason is Brad Thyroff. Brad and I both play in regional tournaments. He is better than me, significantly. The problem, though, is not just that he his better than me, but that literally in every tennis tournament in which he is playing, I keep landing him first round. Tournament after tournament. I just can't catch a break. He goes on to win those tournaments, which is why he is number 1. I keep going down this road again and again. It is not a one way road; it is circular and bitter.

Finally, I sign up for a tournament in Buffalo, New York where the one rule is you can only play if you have never won a tournament. I crush the competition. It is a breeze. It is also the one and only tennis tournament I win until I hit my fifties.

I am 18 years old. I am undefeated in four years of my high school tennis career. We are coming down to the home stretch. Brighton High School, my school, has on the docket Mendon High School. I play 3rd singles (we have a great team, and one of those kids ahead of me is younger than my age bracket but perhaps best in New York State). I should be playing some joe shmoe at Mendon but they cook the books. Who do they put against me at third singles? The best player in the area for my age bracket: Brad Thryoff, the kid who would go on to be the hitting partner for Serena Williams, the GOAT (Greatest Of All Time in women's tennis). I end my high school tennis career with only one loss. This road was circular.

In life, there are some roads that are circular for good or ill, but there are some that thankfully only go in one direction. We are only born once, girls go through menarche once, we go through puberty and grow into full height once, 50% of us go through menopause once, and we die once. Except for the last one, we are generally happy that these are one way roads as their endings often mark a milestone in development.

Not every woman I know is thrilled to go through menopause, but I would say a high percentage are. The classics of Chinese medicine talk about life stages following certain yearly cycles that are different between men and women. Men age in 7 year increments and women age in 8. Menarche and menopause, while in reality are very variable for each individual as to timing, according to the classics, they generally follow specific increments of time. Most of what I have read in the classics, I think are spot on, but I feel these classical factoids do not truly stand the test of time, especially since menarche is occurring at younger and younger ages around the world. We live in a highly estrogenic world where estrogenic plastic makes up our clothes and fills our food and water with microplastics. This is likely why menarche is earlier.

Menopause can also be very variable with some women starting it in the forties and others even as late as their fifties. There are many things I have been able to reverse with my clinical work for short or long periods of time, but one thing I have never been able to do is reverse menopause – to everyone' relief, including my own (imagine revering menopause by accident).

In recent years, I have focused more and more on hormones and their functional activity in the body. Only recently, do I feel I have figured out this interesting puzzle as to why this road is a one way trek. I believe the eggs in the ovaries directly produce the hormones that keep the menstrual cycle persisting and that when enough eggs have been released, there is a critical threshold of a hormone that no longer is maintained in circulation, resulting in menopause.

This is not exactly rocket science as we do know that removal of the ovaries results in immediate menopause at any age. However, I do not feel science has yet identified what specific hormone the eggs are making that maintain the cycle. I feel that is likely to be androstenedione, the same hormone I associate with hot flashes when it is out of balance and with libido and sexual pleasure – when produced in glands not in the ovaries.

Women are often given bio-identical progesterone in order to create a lining when artificial cycles are restored to the body, but as soon as you stop the progesterone, the lining also stops being created. I believe the androstenedione is a deeper level hormone that must be maintained at a certain level in the blood for all of the elements of the menstrual cycle to continue. Perhaps time will tell if I'm correct. I'll be the first to tell you, in this I could be wrong.

The deeper issue, however, is that not all aspects of aging are uninvited guests. I, for one, am happy to **not** go through puberty a second time. I appreciate certain aspects of the aging process. Aging is not our enemy. Aging with enduring and compounding suffering is. Fortunately, those roads, which feel very circular to us, often have off ramps. But it is best to just plain never go on those bumpy roads to begin with, if you can help it.

Key Takeaways:

- Menopause is likely generated by hormones produced by eggs in the ovaries reducing below a threshold when enough eggs have been shed
- Androstenedione, the same hormone that can cause hot flashes and plays a role in libido is likely the factor in keeping women's cycles persisting

A Twisting Tale Of Joint Torquing

I am 18 years old. In my head, I am a scholar athlete. I feel prime in every way. In Maslow's hierarchy of needs, I feel I have reached peak. My ego is so tall, I am telling possible young suitors that I am not interested in their advances even before they ask. I am a ding dong – but I haven't yet gotten the message. The world is my oyster. I feel I can do anything, be anything, and dream anything.

I am 18 years old. I have started Swarthmore College, surrounded by scholars and athlete scholars. I likely have Lyme disease. While I have made a few buddies, I feel like no one I reach out to wants to be my friend, like I'm radioactive. People who say they will meet up with me at certain times at certain places don't bother to show up and never acknowledge plans were made. I am fatigued all day every day. I am flu-like every weekend. I am full of angst. I am depressed. I am lonely and feel abandoned. I am a ding dong, but this time, I have received the message.

Torquing is usually not a good thing when it comes to the spirit but it is arguably even worse if it happens to parts of the body not meant to pull, twist, or bend – or, at least, in the direction it is pointing. Torquing means suffering. The most common place to see this is at the toes, where one toe bends over another. Sometimes there is stretching in odd directions of a digit or more – perhaps without overlap but nevertheless problematic. Most people will suffer toe torquing. No one is talking about this.

The spine is another common location of chronic torquing. Everyone has heard of scoliosis, but then there are also dowager's humps curving the upper spine and even chronic folding of the spine forward in an uncontrollable bowing position. Severed ligaments and/or tendons can be causes of these issues, but in my experience these are more rare. Large swellings of bones or significant bone spurs can generate torques and bends, but often these are just not large enough to create significant issues. The main problem, however, is something people just don't ever think about – a build up of foreign fibers that constantly pull on tissues in errant ways due to pathogens we don't even acknowledge are infecting the body.

Swollen Bones And Bone Spurs

Swollen bones large enough to create obvious shape changes in the body often are the result of Alternaria fungus infecting the bone marrow of the bone. When infected internally with a pathogen that increases estrogen and progesterone locally, the bone will swell over time. The good news is that I have seen time after time that if you clear the Alternaria, this swelling completely reverses.

You will know that a bone is a factor in torquing if there is an obviously swollen bone somewhere along the pathway of the joint. Often this happens at the metatarsal bone heads at the feet to cause torquing of toes or at the metatarsal heads of the hands to cause torquing of the fingers. This also can cause dowager's humps and severe back scoliosis or bending.

A diagnosis of arthritis is common with these issues as bones will clearly be swollen in basic x-rays. However, to doctors this means this is a badge to carry for life with symptomatic care only. In my paradigm, these issues are mediated by fungus infecting the bones that can be remediated.

Besides repetitive activities that cause bone shape changes due to accommodation to the activity itself (super rare in Western societies), the one and only "go-to" for me for a bone spur is Stachybotrys mold. This kind of mold is most known for its association with "Black Molds" but Stachybotrys is a wide class known as a Genus whereas the Black Molds are species within this class, which is to say that are plenty of Stachybotrys infections that are not Black Molds. Nevertheless, any bone spurs in the body is a sign of a chronic or recurring exposure to mold whether in one's home, vehicle, or work environment. A bone spur is a five alarm fire that you need to find and clear any such fungus in your living or working environments because continued exposure will lead to more and more bone spurs, with an increasing likelihood over time of one leading to frozen shoulder or worn down ligaments and tendons to the point of painful injury. If you have a bone spur, you can't just clear fungus with the protocols in this book as you absolutely must find the source of the mold and clear it or else everyone in that same environment will be prone to recurring illnesses, likely chronic sinus and/or breathing issues, and pain – not to mention a wide range of chronic negative emotions.

That said, follow the normal fungal protocols, as these will be protective and can reverse many aspects of bone swelling. This won't cause bone spurs to melt away, unfortunately. It is important to exercise regularly if you have bone spurs as there needs to be some force that can help them whittle down. The caveat to this, of course, is if a ligament or tendon is being damaged by the activity – in which case surgery may be the only remaining option. This is a shame, since it can be very easy to melt away bone spurs with my method. There simply are no great self-care tools out there that can offer the same kind of quick relief.

There are spongy devices that can be used to divide the toes from overlapping. This is purely symptomatic relief and does nothing to solve the root issue. You might consider using these mechanisms if they help you stand and walk without pain. But don't use these and neglect the deeper issue that is fundamental to the problem.

"Ivy Plants"

There are pathogens that can infect the body that I call "Ivy Plant Array" as there is not just one (hence "array") but they include species such as poison ivy. Once in the body, their cells surprisingly can continue to survive and grow. This concept is unheard of in Western medicine and if you mention it to your primary care physician, I will assuredly be laughed at. However, I live in a world of open-mindedness and especially when it comes to infectious organisms, which were around for 2 billion years before multi-cellular organisms showed up and are so much more advanced than anyone understands. It is actually quite shocking. If you are wondering why in the 21st century there is still so much physical suffering, a good deal as to why is that we live in a microbiol soup and that the microbes are completely under appreciated for their inherent cleverness.

Ivy Plant Array are organisms that act like ivy plants in that they use fibers that they produce to anchor to a tissue in the body and then they extend their infection from that anchor to another location where they will anchor next. If you ever tried to pull an ivy plant off of wood, you no doubt struggled. The fibers they use to anchor their tissues to the wood are incredibly strong and persistent. So strong, in fact, you no doubt found yourself pulling off the plant while the anchoring fibers remained attached to the wood.

Many "warts" people have are actually the anchoring fibers of these organisms, where you are seeing on the outside only the impression these are leaving from the bulky anchor inside of your body. While some warts are created by Human Papilloma Virus as we have been taught, which is excess collagen, elastin, and fibrin from the HPV pathogen creating the hardened skin, often enough, however, warts are from Ivy Plant Array. Sometimes, they are from anaerobic fungal pathogens that produce fibrous threads called mycelium.

Ivy Plant Array creates fibers that extend far from the last anchor to create a new anchor elsewhere. This means there can be long fibrous pathways created by these organisms. Once a minimum of two anchors exists, there is the possibility that the tissues to which these anchors have attached start to be pulled towards each other over time. If one anchor is at the end of a toe and another is at the top of that toe's metatarsal bone, then the toe will be pulled up and back, for instance. However, if the second anchor is on the adjacent toe's metatarsal bone head, the toe will be pulled towards that adjacent toe, leading to touching or possibly overlapping of the toes, which can be uncomfortable.

Any kind of persistent torquing of tissues such as twisted vertebra can be from this same phenomenon. Extensive bowing of the back and scoliosis can have this as its root.

Unless an anchor is released from its attached tissue, the torquing and bending of tissues from this phenomenon will unfortunately continue. Some therapies such as myofacial release and rolfing, which I would constitute as uncomfortable, can sometimes stretch or break these fibers and this can help relieve the pulling action.

The unfortunate news is that there are no great "go to" remedies for Ivy Plant Array as these are not bacterial pathogens nor anaerobes nor fungi. There is no grandmother's wisdom that I am aware of to melt away these fibers. There are homeopathic remedies for poison ivy and perhaps these might help, though I have never tried them. Instead, I recommend manual manipulation as I mentioned above, which does not solve the infection side of things, only the fibrous impacts. I will also say that you should aggressively work to clear all warts you find on you as this may be a way to help detach visible attachments of these organisms. Other attachments will be deeper than you can see or treat and so these are the low-hanging fruit of this issue, so you certainly should take advantage of it. In terms of warts, I am more concerned about plantar warts (large and singular) compared to common warts (many tiny warts around a small area) as being potentially Ivy Plant Array attachments.

Perhaps by version 2 of this book, after I have had a chance to talk with other people around the community who have encountered similar issues, there might be more self-care advice about Ivy Plants. Any remedies that dissolve foreign fibers, and anti-microbiols that kill these types of cells.

I recommend prevention as best you can by wearing a mask when exposed to forest fire smoke. The reason I say this is that often forest fires burn up poison ivy and other ivys and their cells are redistributed by the smoke far and wide, including into the human body. Wearing an N95 or its equivalent mask at times of exposure to this smoke is protective. If you are an avid gardener, wear closed toe shoes (not sandals or flip flobs) and gloves especially when weeding. Consider masking when weeding as well. I can just see the eyes rolling over these suggestions. That's fair. I will say, however, my largest population of patients with torquing and twisting issues are gardeners. No lie; no joke. You could say that is just correlation and those people who have the time to garden are perhaps older and more likely to have torquing issues. I am simply asserting that the gardening is a risk factor and you can take it from there.

Key Takeaways:

- Torquing and twisting of tissue is common as a byproduct of infectious disease
- Fungal pathogens and Ivy Plant Array are the main culprits, though the mechanics by which they cause bending and twisting is entirely different

Sinewy, Thinning Membranes, And Dry

It is 2004 and it is also 2007. I am at the hospital holding a newborn. I am crying like a baby myself, my heart is so full and I feel so relieved. Within days and weeks of birth, they are full of their mother's milk and plump. My eldest's cheeks are so full, my dad starts calling her Winston Churchill. Each is soft and warm, with the most gentle skin. They are delightful little furnaces heating up my chest as their bulbous arms dangle from our baby bjorn. Except for the sleeplessness, the crying, and the rare blow out diarrhea, they are my plump little delights warming up my soul.

The aging body undergoes many changes from adolescents to aged. When you look at young people, their skin has moisture but is taut, their subcutaneous tissues are plump, and while they can have issues with dry skin and other similar issues (ie. cradle cap, constipation, eczema, and more) they have a shine and glow to their skin. At the far end of aging, the skin, by contrast, tends to be paper thin and easily broken. There is much less vibrance and hardly any glow. The skin is not taut but wrinkly. People who make it into their nineties and beyond are often thin and sinewy. "Sinewy" means you can easily see the tendons.

A few issues account for this. First, there is a loss of bone that no longer can keep the soft tissues taut. This is the main factor along with the amount of stress one has been subjected to over a lifetime that accounts for all of the wrinkles. I have talked extensively about factors that cause bone loss in the chapter on Bone Softening. Stress is a harder issue to address, as by the time one reads this book, no doubt a person with high stress has already borne the brunt of its impact. There are supplements one can take to help reduce ongoing, enduring, or high stress that includes SAMe (which not everyone can tolerate) and Ashwaganda. Some people simply do not make enough MAO and COMT enzymes for genetic reasons, in which case stress swims around their systems endlessly. I am an Ashkanazi Jew and I believe this runs heavily in Ashkanazi genetics – but I have seen the same phenomenon in my Asian patients, far from the Ashkanazi heritage, and so feel these genetic propensities likely date back to the earliest ages of humankind. The more stress that swims in one's circulation, the more wrinkling as one ages. I also encourage people to adopt life style stress relievers, which I think are much more important than supplements. I believe cardiovascular exercising almost every day of the year is very important and especially important for those who swim in stress due to family, work, or genetics. Exercise supplants the need for COMT and MAO as the stress hormones are broken down through other mechanisms.

It is almost universal that people as they age start to show their blood vessels through their skin. The main culprit here is the same one that can increase urinary incontinence in people as they age or vaginal pain with sex due to wall thinning. Pregnenolone is an essential hormone for tissues as, in my experience, it encourages nitric oxide secretion. Nitric oxide is a capillary and small blood vessel dilator. In a tissue with normal amounts of pregnenolone, tissues are appropriately full of blood due to this dilation effect. When pregnenolone is too high, there is too much dilation, and tissues swell up with blood. Many diseases and imbalances have this imbalance as a major contributing factor, as there are all kinds of mechanics involved where one swollen tissue impinges on another which can occlude vessels that should otherwise be open, press on nerves, bulge organs or the skin, and so forth. The more universal issue with aging, however, is too little pregnenolone leading to too little blood vessel dilation, which will cause affected tissues to not be sufficiently full of blood, causing thinning. This can happen at the urinary sphincter, leading to leakage. This can happen to the vaginal wall, leading to pain with intercourse. This can lead to the skin, leading to a sinewy look as the skin thins and the blood vessels and tendons beneath them show more prominently.

It is at this moment in time that I will remind you that earlier in this book I mentioned how maligned cholesterol is and how we are forced to keep it under control mainly due to the Standard American Diet. Cholesterol is actually the precursor to pregnenolone and if we become deficient in cholesterol (ie. due to taking too high a dose of statins, then all major hormones become deficient, including pregnenolone). This is also one of those places in this book where I have to remind you that while I am a practitioner of Chinese medicine, I am not YOUR medical doctor. If you are concerned that you are getting low in pregnenolone as you combat cholesterol, you should absolutely discuss this with your primary care physician. I do not advocate changing medicines on your own, as this can be dangerous.

All that said, there are reasons why your pregnenolone might be low that have absolutely nothing to do with pharmaceutical drugs meant to control cholesterol. As I have explained, mirror image hormones are often created by organisms in order to trick the body into thinking it has a hormone when in fact its isomer (mirror image) does not in any way behave similarly to the original. The isomers, chelates, and isomer chelates of pregnenolone do not cause nitric oxide secretion and therefore do not dilate blood vessels in a healthy way. These isomers promote thinning of tissues. There are two problems here. First, there are organisms chronically infecting that are generating these isomers. Second, the body does not have natural enzymes necessary to break down these isomers and so they can persist indefinitely if not immediately cleared by the liver. Unfortunately, every category of pathogen can create isomers of pregnenolone, which means there is also no "one and done" cure to stopping the production of these isomers in the body. I therefore, recommend that you follow the chapter on Your Reverse-Aging Calendar to regularly clear pathogens, which over time will address potential contributors of pregnenolone isomers to the body. I will also add that one of the diets that has repeatedly been promoted by science as a healthy diet is the Mediteranean diet, which is high in healthy fats. These fats include healthy cholesterols which can convert into pregnenolone. I recommend eating more aligned with this diet for many reasons, but it may just help in keeping the tissues from thinning out, as an added benefit.

Lastly, I want to address dryness as a factor of blood and circulation. It is common in my practice for people to show up with cracked skin in the hands/fingers/feet/toes and all I have to do is improve circulation in order for this to fully heal. There is a clear relationship with dryness and circulation – not just for circulatory benefits, but because better circulation means more blood, which is full of fluid called plasma and also the great gift of oxygen, which fuels all cellular functions via the Krebs Cycle in the mitochondria generating a molecule called ATP.

As people age, they don't just tend to have worse and worse circulation, the blood itself starts to run low. The bone marrow is hot in nature naturally and the bones are cold. This Yin/Yang relationship generates all Five Elements, which results in the bone marrow being one of the most productive tissues of the body in generating blood and energy that gets distributed head to toe. As we age, the Fire Qi in the bone marrow can become weak as the Water Qi in the bones melts off and migrates into it as part of natural bone reductions discussed earlier in the book. This natural battery of the body becomes much less productive, resulting in less blood creation. All it takes is one bad incident of excessive bleeding, and this can create a negative spiral in a person's vitality and life force. It is very common for my very elderly patients to suffer a bleed that cannot be isolated as to its location, leading to the need for blood transfusions. This is usually quite a red flag. [As a quick aside, sometimes these bleeds have to do with low pregnenolone leading to thinner blood vessel walls.]

It is therefore important to eat more Fire Qi foods as one ages. Of these, the most important is cinnamon, the hottest food in our diet that is hot enough to get into the blood vessels and therefore also the bone marrow. It is very important to eat more cinnamon. This improves circulation and is therefore tangentially important for skin dryness. As we say, however, nothing is good in excess. So, follow the calendar periods when cinnamon is recommended in the Calendar at the end of this book for the most ideal times to increase cinnamon according to seasons and yearly cycles. Other Fire Qi foods include black tea, green tea, coffee, and dark chocolate.

Key Takeaways:

- People wrinkle from bone loss and stress, both of which can be addressed to some degree (see the chapter on Bone Softening)
- Pregnenolone is key in maintaining full skin. It is made from cholesterol and therefore statins might be an issue in thinning

tissues

- The Mediteranean diet offers healthy fats as a way to maintain healthy pregnenolone
- Dryness is often a byproduct of poor circulation and not enough blood. Cinnamon, taken according to a seasonal schedule, may help in avoiding dryness by maintaining healthy circulation and warming the bone marrow

Emotional Mine Fields: Loss And Passion Pits

It is 1994, I move part time to Hamilton, NY. It is 1995, I move to Media, PA. It is 1997, I move to Seattle. It is 1999, I move to Boston. It is 2004, I move to Frederick, MD. It is 2008, I move to Rochester, NY. Each time I move, I lose my community. Each time I move, my wife and I start all over. It is a challenge – more so for my extroverted wife who needs people more than me. Actually, more so for me because as an introvert, it is very hard to meet anyone. Each move, we find ourselves mourning the community we just lost in order to jump into this next adventure.

Naturally, we instinctively know that during our caccoon phase in a new location, the best thing we can do are Sunday morning drives. We drive up and down, left and right, North, South, East, and West. We don't know at the time that we are building our Fire Qi and protecting our spirits through this act of discovery and experimentation. Some places turn out easier than others for building community. But even easier isn't easy. And yet, we instinctively know movement, motion, curiosity, and discovery are essential for our emotional cores.

Everyone has to face hardships in life regardless of socio-economic circumstances. We all have emotions and while some people are better than others in regulating their psychic spaces, there are major emotional hits that one will face – all but guaranteed.

Loss

I have talked earlier about sadness and grief as a facet of life but I feel I should elucidate further about loss. We all must suffer loss. It is the darkest note in this symphony. It is the most tormenting and draining of life's experiences. I have spoken about the dissipating nature of grief when it comes to one's energy. But I have not spoken about the empty space it leaves within us which is in many ways a separate phenomenon from the grief itself.

The people around us bring us joyful memories and companionship. We also carry some of their energy within us. When people die, as an energy intuitive, I can feel this energy get pulled out of me – which speaks to the fact that loss is real loss. It is not just a figure of speech, but we lose energy and have more void within us when a family member or friend dies. We feel drained because we are in some ways drained of an energy that was within us bringing us solace even when far and away in physical distance.

In areas known as "Blue Zones" where people have been found to live much longer than most areas of the world, one clear factor in these areas according to those who study them, is a sense of community. In some communities, people age with the very same people with whom they went to elementary school – meaning there is a richness and depth in those relationships that few people in my country of the United States, where moving from city to city across this giant landmass is very much the norm, do not usually experience.

When you have community, loss can be more easily absorbed and when you are isolated, you feel it far more acutely. In many religious traditions, there are processes by which the community surrounds and supports its members when they experience loss, as a way to buoy the spirit and to help, where possible, fill the empty spaces. In the era that I wite this book, however, we have fewer of these communities. Far fewer people affiliate with a religious institution and more people find themselves using smartphones and televisions to fill their hours that previously would have been filled with face-to-face experiences with others.

I do not believe religious institutions need to fill this role of community, but they are good at it, with hundreds if not thousands of years of religious and cultural practice well honed to address those who survive another's passing. I do believe, however, that people need to have face-to-face time with others as succor for the soul. I say this as an introvert who has a fair aversion to public gatherings. I also write this as the Sars-CoV-2 (Covid 19) pandemic just ravaged a lot of social intelligence by way of social isolation necessary for survival. Many of us found it easier to be alone than to be with others after our social fabric atrophied.

I am also not saying that people should be social exclusively to protect their spirit for the periods of time in which they experience loss. Obviously, one should be social to experience the myriad benefits that come from connection and the joys of smiling and laughing with others. This social fabric is important. We can't try to make Blue Zones just be joining book clubs. We can, however, understand that these group activities are filling parts of our energy spaces that we cannot easily recognize without being unusually attuned to energy. You can be attuned to your heart and emotions and how people make you feel, which should be obvious. Be with people; age with people. It is how we have evolved and it is part of how we make meaning of life's experience.

Passion Pits

The energy of passion is Fire Qi in Chinese medicine, which is fueled by another element called Wood Qi (we call this its "Mother" and the Fire Qi the "child.") You can't have a child without its mother, which means both energies are necessary to have healthy passion. Wood Qi is the energy of flexibility, growth, and change – three factors that reduce as people age. When people grow older, they discover they like what they like and increasingly they reduce even trying something new but keep within certain paths of behavior that within this book I have lovingly called "ruts." The older we get, the deeper the ruts, and the less likely one is willing to move outside these deep ruts to do something unexpected.

Fire Qi is the energy of stimulation, adrenaline, novelty, love, passion, and joy. As we get older, and our ruts deepen, we are less likely to seek out high stimulation experiences – which is precisely opposite to what teenagers are doing, by example. The older one gets, the more likely that companions in life (friends and family) pass away, which is very hard on love, passion, and joy.

The combined "one-two" punch of less change and transformation combined with less stimulation and passion is a tremendous diminishing of light in one's life. Fire Qi is the energy of light. Wood Qi and Fire Qi when combined generate an energy we call Yang, or heat. People are in danger of more physical cold as well as emotional cold as life turns more inward, more Yin.

It is my belief that Fire Qi is a major contributor for our aging and when it diminishes, this is an actual danger on a "spiritual" level, however you might want to define spiritual. I am defining it here as meaning a danger to the propelling energy that sends you forward into more life with more experiences. When enough Fire Qi diminishes, the spiritual flame extinguishes.

One way that I have designed Fire Qi into my aging process is to always plan my next anticipated adventure even as I am finishing up the present one like a procession of pearls on a chain. I am currently in my working years, and so this shows up as always knowing where I will be traveling to next even as my current adventures are being enjoyed. I think of this as a carrot to always keep my eyes on. One adaptation of this model for those who are retired is to always think of the next friend or family you are going to visit, and be willing to push through any physical impediment and/or traveling discomfort to get there (as needed).

Travel is both Wood Qi and Fire Qi. It is change and getting out of one's ruts (Wood Qi) and it is the newness and stimulation that is part and parcel of an adventure (Fire Qi). I am a huge advocate for travel, but one can get Fire Qi and Wood Qi through other means.

Wood Qi foods are sour in taste. Anything sour you eat, has some Wood Qi in it. Limes and lemons are the highest in Wood Qi. Fire Qi foods include dark chocolate, cinnamon, black tea, coffee, and green tea. If it speeds up your heart or makes you feel happy, it has Fire Qi in it.

Wood Qi athletics involve back and forth activities such as swimming or any other activity with laps. Fire Qi athletics are on the move in new locations over time, which includes walking outdoors, hiking, running, and cycling. I will note that walking outdoors in nature trails and forests combines Wood Qi and Fire Qi, making nature bathing a particularly powerful way to age with these energies.

It is my belief that you need to protect your spirit as you age as if it is a candle flame that strong winds can extinguish. You need to be active in the defense of your spirit. And, in this case, I mean you need to actively defend your Wood Qi and Fire Qi. It is very easy to sit in your favorite chair, watch your favorite shows, eat ice cream, and let that flame extinguish itself by doing nothing to protect it. In fact, most people do this. Now, there is nothing wrong with sitting in your favorite chair and watching your favorite show and even eating ice cream from time to time. But it is easy to sink into those ruts and not get out of them – so very very easy not to travel, not to visit friends or families, not to seek out stimulation that might include cold temperatures or that activate achy joints.

As an aside, I will note that Wood Qi is about flexibility and inasmuch, it also relates to joints – where most people experience increasing stiffness and tightness over time. Stretching is a hugely important way to keep your joints flexible and, you guessed it, this increases Wood Qi as well. My moniker: "use it or lose it" refers to your joints. The less you move a joint, the more likely it stops being one. This is one reason I feel dance is perhaps the most important exercises that most people give up rather than adopt as they age. Dance moves every joint and it is actually another amazing Wood Qi and Fire Qi exercise.

How does this all relate to happiness, joy, and passion? On the one hand, the less you can move your body, the less joy you will have as it limits your range of options in life. Secondly, energy is energy and if you build it up by dancing, that same energy builds up emotionally as happiness and joy. On a scientific level, you can certainly point to enkephalins, endorphins, and dopamine as playing a Fire Qi role that connects dance and nature bathing with happiness. However, you want to explain it, moving your body is one of the most important ways to protect your spiritual flame.

But what if you cannot move your body? Then read. Reading is like walking outdoors, it comes with newness, the unexpected, twists and turns. Which means the most important part of the body to protect if you are limited in your physical mobility are your eyes. But even if your eyes go, you can listen to audio books very easily in the modern era. Find authors that you absolutely love. Love is Fire Qi. There are many ways to cultivate it.

Key Takeaways:

- Maintaining community is essential, even for the introverts among us
- Protecting Wood Qi and Fire Qi via diet, activities, future planning, and intentionally busting through one's ruts is essential for protecting one's spiritual flame
- Travel, hiking in nature, and dance are three examples of activities that protect the spirit and when these are impossible books and audio books can also build life force

Mental Clouds

It is April 1991. I am flying back from college for a holiday weekend from Philadelphia to Rochester. It is a short flight, but the weather is terrible and the turbulence is tremendous. Later in life, I become a more Zen flyer but even if my Zen self was in that plane, my palms would be sweaty and holding tight to the seat railing for dear life. We end up circling Rochester for an extra hour waiting for a window to land.

The plane starts its descent. We pop out of the clouds into a very dark and rainy scene. The clouds are low to the ground and so when we emerge from this cumulous blanket, we are already close to the ground. The plane is preparing for landing. We are over the runway when suddenly the nose of the plane does the opposite of my expectations, instead of pointing downward, it suddenly points up. Instead of descelerating, the plane starts accelerating with significant G force. My mind stops working as I cannot make sense of the situation. My knuckles are white, I am holding so tightly to the seat handles. We pop back into the clouds and we're back to circling around Rochester. The kind man with gentle eyes next to me demonstrates no alarm. He notes mine, however. He explains that we experienced an "aborted landing" which can happen when a pilot feels the cross winds are too strong and it would be dangerous to the plane and passengers. Thirty minutes later, we attempt another landing and the winds have died down, the descent is surprisingly calm and peaceful. We touch ground smoothly. The passengers cheer. I am literally and figuratively shook, but cheering along with them, making sure to thank the pilots as we pass them as I'm steered off the plane.

Sometimes the mind is calm and we fly through our consciousness smoothly, but at other times, there are dark clouds and turbulence. This is normal and natural. There are even times when we fly with minds that are not quite right, not catching every detail or understanding every situation. This can be normal and natural as well. In my senior year of high school, on a fine Spring day, I walked down the hallway only to have my field of vision shrinking into a tunnel. I wasn't sure the circumstances but thought perhaps it was best to sit down before I fainted. It was the start of the flu and a good example of the mental airship losing its tether and this being a normal part of the human experience.

During Covid, I noticed people's memories were far worse than normal. I also found my own intellect not nearly as sharp and my memory, which historically was particularly acute, significantly worsened – especially the immediate months after having a bout with the virus myself. Things deteriorated for me internally though I am not sure anyone but my wife would have noticed a drop in mental acuity. But *I* certainly did and it was alarming. Losing memory is a frightful thing – and most people are afraid of Alzheimer's as most people have had family members or friends experience some form of dementia. Early in my work, I found it was common for infectious organisms to increase sugars in the body as a way of attacking the lymphatic system. These sugars stagnate the lymphatic fluid. In most of the body, this causes fatigue, but in the head, it generates brain fog. I have found other molecules can have a similar impact, such as C-reactive protein, a common Covid toxin, and one of the pathways by which it causes mental confusion.

High blood sugar is obviously not just relegated to viral toxins. Adult onset Type II Diabetes is one of the most common byproducts of the Standard American Diet. It is not just that we eat a tremendous amount of white sugar, which is both delicious and poisonous to our systems, starches removed of their fibers such as white breads and white rice make their sugars freely available during digestion and are main culprits (along with the over-consumption of red meat) in raising blood sugar in most people.

C-reactive protein is a blood vessel inflammation marker. Cardiovascular disease is one of the topmost killers and another common byproduct of the Standard American Diet, which is usually high in animal fats – not the only cause of arteriorsclerosis, but certainly a significant contributor.

There are many things you can do to reduce your risk factors for diabetes and cardiovascular disease, such as exercising and eating healthy. One suggestion I have is to eat vegetarian one month and vegan one month within every 12 months of a year. This is not a perfect replacement for eating a Meditteranean diet all year, which is more protective. But to take 60 days a year off all animal fats can help to cleanse your blood vessels of debris and is better than driving full steam into the future with the diet you inherited from people who did not know anything about anything about diet and the body, and simply wanted to survive the brutally cold Winters (no offense to our ancestors intended). I eat sugar in my coffee and occasional treats. I eat lean white meat regularly. I do not eat a Meditteranean diet, even though it has been well studied to be the most optimal diet for aging. That said, I do eat vegetarian/pescetarian (eating fish and eggs) one month and vegan one month intentionally during the year. I also intentionally eat a very varied diet inspired by many nationalities all week long as well as varied across the months to ensure variability of nutrients – and also to expand the joy of my heart. Will I live to be 100? Not likely. Will I suffer fewer dangerous impacts from my diet than if I ate the SAD diet day after day ad nauseum? I hope so. I know I live with some risk. The point is one should not just eat oblivious to the risks – but self-aware that diet is perhaps the biggest input to your aging comfort.

Alzheimer's is sometimes called Type III Diabetes as it is thought that it is a sign of sugar dysregulation with the brain. The inflammatory impact of high blood sugar on blood vessels that go to the brain reduces their blood flow just as much as it does to the toes, fingers, feet, and hands – you can think of each of these as the distal ends of circulatory distribution, which makes them the most vulnerable. It is known that cardiovascular disease and Alzheimer's have a direct relationship. While the genes in your DNA are far less within your capacity to change, your diet is well within your control as to what you eat or do not eat. Therefore, what you eat are the "control nobs" you can turn for optimum influence over your aging brain.

Intermittent Fasting can also be beneficial to the mind as it activates genes that cleanse you on a cellular level, but the contents of what you eat when you eat even on a "fasting" diet still matters.

DHEA And Covid

When the pandemic Sars-Cov-2 (Covid) struck, I found myself for close to three years in an endless loop treating the same issues with my patients. It was exhausting and I am not surprised that so many healthcare practitioners burnt out and left medical fields as it was both relentless and, honestly, boring on a professional level. I mean no insult to anyone who lost family members to the disease when I say it was boring. Imagine a general practitioner who loves solving complex problems and being stuck in a loop for three years only afforded the same singular problem to treat again and again? I hope you see what I mean? Certainly, people did have other issues, which kept me intellectually in the game, but there was a constant dull hum of the same problem with the same symptoms. It was relentless.

One of those symptoms that kept coming up was memory loss. As I said, I personally experienced this as well. On the one hand, there was the memory loss of simply being much less stimulated living in a world with far fewer options out of the house. But in short time, society started to percolate with activity and more stimulation was available. There was memory loss from having to keep in the back of one's mind the need to bring a mask, wear a mask, be grossed out by people breathing on you, thinking about the air as a contaminated space, thinking about surfaces that were touched by hundreds of other people, etc. Some people cared more about this and some cared less. For many, however, it ate a part of the mind enough to keep out just enough other more varied stimulation to weaken some mental acuity.

But the biggest issue was the virus itself. It produces toxins that are bad for memory. I mentioned the C-reactive protein earlier, but it also produced something that I feel was more insidious and far worse, which were isomers (remember, these are mirror images to the actual shape of a molecule) of DHEA.

DHEA is a hugely important molecule for memory AND consciousness, it turns out. Yes, it plays an important role as a precursor to androgens which are precursors for testosterones which are precursors to estrogens. Not having enough proper shapes of DHEA will completely mess up this entire cascade of essential hormones for both men and women. More importantly, however, I feel DHEA itself is the most important molecule for memory directly (outside of magnesium) and plays a direct, essential role in other cognitive functions including executive functioning (knowing which steps go in which order in order to accomplish basic as well as complex tasks).

One very common Covid symptom was disruption of taste and smell which is mediated by the olfactory nerve. In my work, I have come to see that the olfactory nerve extends from the nose, to the "third eye" level of the cerebrum and then straight back through the entire cerebrum, very much in parallel with the optic nerve that is an inch or so above it. I have come to see that the olfactory nerve plays a fundamental role in memory recall, having branches that go into areas of the brain that relate to memories about people we know and other branches where we hold words and names, by way of example. Disruption of this nerve is highly problematic for memory, it turns out. And, as I said, Covid prefers to infect this particular cranial nerve.

Which is to say, Covid messed with people's brains in a very specific way that may very well explain why on a society level across almost every country on every continent, there was great difficulty in people agreeing on how to handle the crisis of an infectious pandemic – we weren't cognitively at our best. In this regard, I am just speculating. But on a professional level, I found that if I focused on helping my patients restore the proper shapes of DHEA in their systems, they improved dramatically in their reported post-Covid memory loss. DHEA is not the only important molecule for activating the olfactory nerve and its recall functions – but it happens to be a very important one and one that can be supplemented over-the-counter (along with magnesium).

In my work, I clear the isomers to help facilitate this. However, anyone can benefit from DHEA supplementation who is suffering from cognitive changes, loss of executive functioning, memory loss, low motivation (sign of low androgens), low testosterone, and low estrogen. Obviously, it is not a cure all for all complaints. It is also important to note that the brain is a complex system and DHEA isomers, high sugars, and C-reactive protein are by far not the only factors that can go wrong that can lead to cognitive and memory complaints. However, they might just be factors that matter for you. For those who wish to supplement with DHEA, I recommend doing so for 30 days. I am not one of those people who think you should go on a supplement forever and the problem with DHEA is that it will increase feelings of angst and brooding if you are on it too long. We say in Chinese medicine: "nothing in excess." Balance is more important than persistence. 30 days is enough to know if it helped you. If it did, great! If it didn't, move on to other ideas. This is similar to why I recommend 30 day stints with dietary changes. You will get benefits from this, but there are also costs from eating any diet too long. People who eat vegan have to be thoughtful about protein consumption, for instance. People who eat macrobiotic tend to get dry. People who eat keto diets have to worry about cholesterol. There are costs to every choice. When you make a choice, you should know the costs and be mindful about their impacts.

Dementia

Obviously, developing dementia is a major concern people have as they age. There are three essentials for memory: 1. The ability to focus, 2. Memory formation, and 3. Memory recall. Interruption of any of these three will result in dementia if the impact is severe and not-reversible. The optic nerve has an area in it essential for executive functioning that plays a role in mental focus along with the anterior amygdala juncture with the thalamus. Memory formation is generated in an area between the optic nerve and olfactory nerve that includes the inferior hypothalamus. Memory recall relates to the olfactory nerve. In many ways, memories are like star maps that when given light, shine a light across the entire brain – invoking the auditory pathways for sounds, the visual pathways for images, the amygdala for emotions, and more.

The key to avoiding dementia is to keep the brain active. One of the great mistakes people make is to think of their retirement as a time to stop exercising the mind when in fact, this is perhaps the most important time in your life to be making sure as many mental bells go off around your star maps as possible. Learning a new language is thought to be one of the most powerfully productive ways to fend off dementia and, if you take a moment to think about it, this makes sense as words are embodiments of sounds, sights, and feelings and invoke a lifetime of one's own memories.

It is commonly thought that olfactory stimulation is one of the most powerful forces in memory. I now believe it may be helpful to invoke perfumes and smells (something I am actually personally somewhat averse) as a way to exercise the olfactory nerve. Which is to say, visit farmer's markets and spice markets, smell everything for their freshness. Seek out natural perfumes as opposed to chemical ones to exercise the brain.

There are other molecules other than DHEA that aid in focus, memory formation, and memory recall that I have identified that include enkephalins (feel good hormones, ie. invoked through human to pet interactions and individual with family and friend interactions, also acts of self-nurturing such as massage or play), norepinephrine (invoked through exciting, stimulating experiences – and human to human interactions). These cannot be supplemented over-the-counter but you can simply make sure <u>not</u> to "check out" of society but to stay involved with your family and community to activate these hormones.

I will speak more about dementia in the next chapter.

<u>Key Takeaways</u>:

- Common causes of cognitive decline include high sugars, blood vessel inflammatory molecules, and DHEA isomers
- Diet is within the realm of your control and can be thoughtfully changed in short bouts of time to protect you from the dangers of the Standard American Diet (the elephant in the room no one talks about)
- DHEA is perhaps the most important molecule for cognitive function, executive functioning, and memory. You can supplement it, but do not stay on it too long or it generates angst
- Other molecules that help with mental focus, memory formation, and recall (the three facets of memory) can be

boosted by not retiring one's mind when one retires, but by staying involved in one's family and in one's community – as human interaction is key to keeping these flowing

Dementia: A Popping Good Story

My snappy, sharp tongued (sometimes a bit stinging tongued, to be honest) Grandma Lotti is 82. My wife and I are visiting her in Fort Lauderdale, FL. The visit is very lovely. I am chewing candies I only eat at Grandma Lotti's, including delicious chocolate covered espresso beans. All is going well until she looks me in the eyes and tells me that she is going to die next year when she turns 83. I am shocked and alarmed. She seems in good health. "Why?" I ask her. She tells me that none of her family members ever made it to 83. This conversation is burnt into my memory banks.

It is one year later and Lotti doesn't die...physically. But out of nowhere, she develops severe dementia. She actually stays alive for a few more years by the heroic effort of people reminding her to eat. But her mind stopped at the age she anticipated. Was this a self-fulfilling prophecy? Hard to say. But it was heart breaking for us all, nonetheless.

The irreversible loss of attention, memory formation, and/or memory recall is expressed as dementia, which can have many flavors, one of which is well known as Alzheimer's. Western science has spent generations on the wrong paths, wrong problems, wrong medicines and has few tools to help. There are many many theories as to the pathway of its formation but no definitive ones. For a quarter of a century, a major focus has been on tau proteins and amyloid plaques and all of the medicines focused on clearing these have been for naught. If you are in a car graveyard full of smooshed cars, you can't stop the smooshing of cars by removing the smooshed cars. That is just the end result of the process. You have to turn off the car smooshing machine. For decades, medicines have been removing the smooshed cars and this sadly hasn't made a lick of difference.

I believe there are multiple pathways to get to dementia, but I am honing in on some new ideas that are very different. For years, I have focused on clearing infectious organisms from the brain and the most important ones being Bornavirus and Toxoplasma (which always infect together). My professional experience with this has been a slowing down the progression of the disease to a bike ride instead of a rocketship. The progression continued more slowly but was not stopped. Lately, I have turned my focus also towards algae, moss, mildew, and lichen as negative agents.

However, I have found some issues that are not in the Western constructs that need to be explored that are indirectly related to infectious diseases – which I am hoping are the car smooshing machines and not just the debris field left around it.

Balloons And Sponges In The Brain

Cells are meant to be always communicating with their environment. They are designed to intake fluids, electrolytes, hormones and more and also to discharge similar but different factors in a regular flow. This flow is not meant to ever be disrupted as the health of the cells entirely depend on this communication.

There are molecules, however, that can be highly disruptive. Some molecules can turn cells that absorb infiltrates and discharge excretions into one way paths of constant infiltration. Cells of this nature turn from being normal cells into being "spongie." They absorb too much and can even stretch over time. Other cells are simply turned into balloons metaphorically tied off at the end, which means they might not be swelling up, but they are also forming a layer of inflexibility. A single cell behaving in such a manner is not such a big deal. But when too many cells behave in this way, it becomes a tissue-level problem – one that can lead to malfunction of that tissue and can even lead into forms of chronic swelling that can impinge on other tissues, including blood vessels, fluid vessels, nerves, and more. This can happen anywhere in the body and is not selective to the brain – but, yes, it also can happen in the brain.

This process of converting from a healthy cell to one that swells more and more or that is cut off from its environment is mediated by molecules. One important molecule is called zonulin. Zonulin is most well known as the factor that causes leaky gut syndrome as it pries open spaces in between cells that should otherwise not exist. I have found that this molecule and others that behave like this can result in cells and tissues becoming spongie. The body can make zonulin on its own as a reaction to physical trauma. But it is also a fairly common toxin of infectious organisms.

Cortisol is a molecule that causes overstretching of tissues. It can do this external to cells but it can also do this internally as well. We make cortisol via our adrenal glands and other locations of the body but this also is a very common toxin made by infectious organisms. If cortisol gets into cells that are turning spongie, those cells will stretch and stretch and stretch until they can no longer stretch any more at all without popping. But they keep stretching and so – "pop!" Cells can start popping like popcorn throughout tissues, leaving a debris field that white blood cells will need to clean up. In the brain, one byproduct of the brain's immune system is amyloid plaque and tau protein. Cells that pop have popped. That is a permanent loss of that cell. If enough cells pop faster than the body can regenerate them, this results in a net loss of cells, which is bad news and especially if this is happening in parts of the brain important for mental focus, memory creation, and/or memory recall.

An Interventionist Approach

The above is a theory based on my work as an intuitive healer. I can see in plenty of people, including myself when I started, pockets of spongy cells. I can see in my Alzheimer's patients, vast swathes of affected cerebral tissue. As a disease of aging, this looks promising as a pathway that goes from small inconsequential pockets into something larger and very consequential over time based on the actions of infectious organisms that are also increasing their colony sizes over time.

As I said, Bornavirus and Toxoplasma are factors in this process and likely algae and moss as well, but they are not the only ones. A list of pathogens that I know that produce zonulin includes: Clostridium Genus, Staphylococcus, Equine Infectious Anemia Virus, Alternaria, HHV6, HHV7, Bacillus Thuringiensis, Aspergillus, Measles, Giardia, Yeasts (including but not limited to Candida Auris), Anaerobic Pathogens, Cholera, Bartonella, Penicillium, Stachybotrys, Salmonella, Tropheryma Whipplei, Stemphylium Vesicarium, Mumps, and H. Pylori. Of this list, one of my greatest concerns are yeasts. I was focusing on Bornavirus and Toxoplasma all these years, but if I had made the connection with zonulin earlier in my career, I would have focused far more on yeasts because the honest-to-goodness truth is that we are cooking our brains with yeast like we are cooking our bread – full of popping pockets. Which is why much of the self-care calendar in this book is about clearing fungal pathogens and yeast from the body, resetting the clock as much as possible.

If you were to ask me which I would give up first: sugar or yeast, my answer would likely be "no." And I think that is true of most people. It is probably a non-starter. Furthermore, I find yeast in my patients who are totally off yeast in their diets and that is because yeast is so prevalent in our society, it is often ambient in the air (ie. at restaurants and bakeries). It is highly unlikely that most readers of this book would take on a totally no-yeast diet and I am not even making that argument. Instead, I feel periodic de-yeasting is a good enough strategy that might end up helping quite a few people. As you can see from my list of known pathogens that generate zonulin, even if you eradicate yeasts, you can still be chronically infected by a totally different pathogen and this could still have negative consequences.

Another consideration in this process is that of "damaging faster than the body can regenerate." The aging process is wrought with slowdowns in self-repair. As I said earlier, it is thought that circulatory factors affecting the brain play a role in dementia such as arteriosclerosis and high blood sugar induced inflammation. This likely negatively impacts the body's ability to heal from damage and disease. Focusing on improving circulation and maintaining healthy blood sugar is important in keeping the body's ability to heal at its maximum possible regenerative speed. In this regard, eating healthy plus daily cardiovascular exercise are key. Human growth hormone or other medicines (ie. statins, blood thinners) or herbs that help with healthy circulation (ie. cinnamon, vitamin E) may further assist one's rate of rejuvenation by helping maintain circulatory vigor. The absolutely worst thing one can do is to eat lots of sugar and yeast, be sedentary all day, and not engage intellectually and emotionally in life. Don't buy into the image of retirement as a "turn off" time of life. That is a one way ride to brain cellular popcorn.

There is assuredly far more to the story of dementia than I am discussing in this all too short chapter. This is a multi-factorial problem and I only see a small piece of it myself. However, what I do see makes sense of quite a bit of observations about the disease (ie. brian size shrinks tremendously with most forms of dementia). I will update future iterations of this book with new discoveries on this topic, as I am most certain to have them.

Key Takeaways:

- Dementia is likely from damage to tissues due to their cells popping from internal forces, mediated by molecules that are common pathogen toxins
- Periodically clearing yeasts from the body may prove hugely helpful by way of prevention
- Exercise, a healthy diet, and perhaps assistance as necessary in maintaining healthy blood sugar and circulation via medicines or herbs each can help the body's rate of rejuvenation, which likely must also slow down for net brain cell loss over time

Perfringens, Necrosis, & Tumors

It is Autumn 2021. One of my favorite patients of all time just passed away from a rare Covid side effect. She was swallowed up by Q Anon conspiracy theory. She told her husband of 50 years that if he received the vaccine, she would leave him so that she wouldn't have to watch him wither and die from it. The rare symptom was gangrene which she suddenly suffered from without any morbid exposure to extreme elements. First, they had to remove her toes but the infection continued. They removed her foot but the infection deepened. Ultimately, it killed her. Such a wonderful human. As a friend and healer, her loss continues to break my heart.

But it also got me thinking about gangrene...

My dog Tibby has had fantastic teeth but I am noticing the front teeth have suddenly pulverized out of nowhere into half their height. The little bits of tooth remaining are covered in rot. Gangrene is on my mind and so I check her out for it. Low and behold, this is the rot!

Gangrene is caused by Clostridium Perfringens, an anaerobic bacterial pathogens. It produces a massive amount of chelated isomers of 21 deoxycortisol. The normal shape of this molecule is what gives bones and teeth hardness and strength but the chelated isomer does the opposite – it makes bones and teeth soft and brittle, prone to chipping and fracturing. My dog Tibby's teeth are riddled with chelated isomers of 21 deoxycortisol. I clear the Clostridium Perfringens, clear the tiny teeth bits and chips floating around, use my methods to restore the 21 deoxycortisol proper shapes, and within days the rot is entirely gone and the remaining half teeth look white and healthy.

As you can imagine, this got my mind revving. Anyone can experience rotting teeth given the right circumstances. Heroin addicts, for instance, are known for their teeth rot. What if this is a bigger, wider issue?

Indeed, over time I came to discover that Clostridium

Perfringens is in practically everyone but it is far more active with much larger colonies in older people. Most elderly people suffer extreme dental issues that include decay, root canal infections, tooth fractures, and more. This is due to the unhindered proliferation of a bacteria that no dentist would ever consider being resident in their patients' mouths despite the fact that we know human bites are actually very dangerous when they break the skin, with great threat of very dangerous infections that can include gangrene.

Clostridium Perfringens is not solely an oral colonizer. It can get to any tissue of the body, including bone tissue, where it can cause unexpected, rapid bone loss at specific bones or joints (as opposed to systemic massive bone loss such as osteopenia or osteoporosis).

Furthermore, tumors are known to be locations where necrotic tissue is regularly found. At tumors, I find what I call "human-to-human cell fusions" where cells are weirdly bonded (not via the normal orderly, side by side presentation connected via what are called "tight junctions" of connective tissues). This is from necrosis of the cell walls – a process mediated by a sharp influx of chelated isomers of 21 deoxycortisol. Adults tend to get cancers, not children and adults tend to get larger colonies of Clostridium Perfringens. Don't get me wrong, I am not saying all cancers are caused by gangrene from this organism but I am saying no one is looking here at all as a contributing factor. I have worked with cancer patients for over two decades in my career and these are complex problems, often very individual in presentation. One thing I do associate with all cancers, however, is a sense of chaos in one's lived experience where something goes out of control in a way that seems potentially destructive or life shattering. Sometimes these are self-limiting chaotic events and sometimes they are seemingly forever chaotic influences. These chaotic episodes are reflective of and, in my mind, generative of tumors.

In the case of growths in the body, I feel it is important for a person to go through one's life and think about what feels chaotic and out of control and think of real, functional solutions as to how to bring that chaos into order. This is a spiritual level issue. If the chaos is self-limiting already, if it has a clear end-date, then no action is needed if that end date is in the near future. But if the problem is open ended – this is dangerous. It is important to establish a sense of control, if possible. Sometimes that means extricating oneself from a toxic situation. Sometimes it means bringing in others or any number of others until there is a sense of established order where before there was chaos.

When looking at the rot in my dog's mouth, it looks like chaos. The teeth literally disintegrated leaving behind a debris field covered in dangerous looking brown goo. Tumors look chaotic. A single cancerous cell looks chaotic and disordered.

I imagine if you are a Western trained medical practitioner, you will think this is all a bunch of correlation and not causation, a bunch of theoretical bunk. You may be right. I am not saying I know for sure the cause of cancer as a sole practitioner even with two and a half decades of experience behind me – it simply is not enough. Perhaps it is the other way around where the chaos entered the system on a spiritual level after the growths appeared, more as a symptom than a cause. Or perhaps the correlation itself is garbage and this is purely speculation. Fair enough. However, I stick to my perception of my patients. I see chaos and cancer correlate among those whom I have treated. And I find an organism in cancer locations that causes cellular chaos hanging out and necrotizing cell walls, causing cell to cell fusions.

You may recall on our initial conversation in the Softening Bones chapter that I recommended the Anaerobic Bacteria Protocol to clear anaerobic pathogens such as Clostridium Perfringens. I am not saying this will prevent or cure cancer as I have no data to back of that assertion. I tend to work on people after they are diagnosed and not on the prevention side of cancer care. However, my work suggests that regularly clearing anaerobic pathogens may just possibly be protective on some level. I would add to that, daily oral care is super recommended not just to keep your teeth but to also keep Clostridium Perfringens from generating a massive colony in the body from which it can extend elsewhere. Any chip of a tooth, fracture of a tooth, chip of a bone, or fracture of a bone should send you immediately into a new cycle of hyper-oxygenating your system (the Anti-Anaerobe protocol) with nettle tea just in case C. Perfringens is a contributing factor. I will add that I perceive parasites at every tumor as a critical building block of their formation. The Anti-Parasite protocol is therefore presented as crucial preventative care.

Key Takeaways:

- Clostridium Perfringens is a nasty organism that Western doctors don't think is a problem for the average person and yet it likely is one of the most dangerous organisms in most people's regular experience
- It is a factor for teeth and bone chipping and fracture
- It is a likely, completely unrecognized contributing factor in tumor formation
- Regular use of the Anaerobic Bacteria Protocol may prove to protective against serious disease
- The Anti-Parasite Protocol is crucial self-care to as best as possible reduce the danger of tumor formation

Your Body Is Just Relaxin

It is August 1987. I am flying back from Israel with a large group of teenagers with whom I have had an amazing, life changing experience. It is a long plane ride home. I spot one of my friends smiling at me, giggling with her friends, and they are all under a blanket. I sit down to say hello and I find myself under the blanket as well.

I thought we were just going to relax together in a cuddle, but the next thing I am aware of is a hand touching my privates. I am 17; so is she. She is smiling at me. I smile back. The hand is doing more than just touching me down under. Soon, I am feeling very good. And then way too soon, I am feeling far too good. Let's just say that at 30,000 feet, I had an unexpected experience. Does this count as joining the Mile High Club? No idea.

The instant it is over, I am mortified. My underwear is a mess. I am in the middle of a plane. I can't believe that just happened. I run to the bathroom while those under the blanket laugh at my embarrassment and awkwardness.

I return to this memory many times over my life with equal parts horror and equal parts humor. And also, notably, zero regrets – except, perhaps, that I was too mortified and stunned to return the favor.

People talk about relaxing into their elder years without quite meaning it so literally that their bodies become loose, gangly, and dangling off their bones. They go in with the expectation of mental relaxation ("retirement, yes!") with every expectation to retain fitness and the ability to travel extensively in fully functioning bodies only to increasingly become physiologically limp, with lost muscle tone, and a tremendous increase in pains and infirmities. One cause of this is a terrible predisposition for people in my country, the United States, to drive everywhere and not exercise sufficiently especially with weight bearing exercises that keep bones full and muscles strong. I won't rehash my feelings on this as I have written sufficiently enough about this earlier in the book.

However, there is an unexpected secondary reason for the body to lose its tautness – including and perhaps even especially facial skin tightness: relaxin. Relaxin is a hormone that is released in a pregnant women days and weeks leading up to labor that so tremendously increases flexibility, it allows ten pound babies to drop from the abdomen where they are snug down the entire birth canal, which includes passing through a thin tunnel in the cervix that is itself usually much smaller than a wine bottle's cork.

It turns out our bodies do generate the hormone relaxin – both men and women – all throughout our lives, at low levels. Yes, it is possible for our bodies to make too much of it. As you have figured out by now, I tend to focus on infectious organisms as the bigger cause of most of our problems and the fact is that while we make relaxin "endogenously" (by our own bodies), the bigger danger we face in terms of sudden, inexplicable aging, is a sudden, heavy dose of "exogenous" relaxin – pathogen toxins released into our systems by infectious disease.

As of this writing, I do not have a wide list of relaxin producing organisms, but we did just go through a Yin Water Qi/Earth Qi year (according to the 60 year Chinese Medicine astrology calendar), which fueled the growth of Paragonimus, a parasite that is a major producer of relaxin. Paragonimus is considered a "lung fluke." The skin and the lungs are made out of the same energy in Chinese medicine, and we effectively perceive no difference between the two, so it should come as no surprise that Paragonimus also causes skin infections which can show up as cystic acne, sores, pins and needle discomfort rashes, and, most commonly, as unexplained widespread itchiness. I will also find this "gu" (what we call multi-cellular parasites in Chinese medicine) all throughout the body which is to say it might have a propensity for "Yin Metal Qi" tissues such as the lungs and skin, but can infect opportunistically wherever it can reach.

The synaptic junctions are made up of two component parts: neurexin and neuroligin. You can think of these as nerve joints, as these are tied together with connective tissues. Connective tissues for synapses are the same energy as connective tissues for the tight junctions between facial skin cells, and the same energy as connective tissues for tendons and ligaments. Think of relaxin for a moment as I do – not as a hormone, but a purveyor of excess Wood Qi. Wood Qi is the energy that makes up connective tissues, ligaments, and tendons. Wood Qi increases flexibility and excess Wood Qi causes hyper-flexion, leading to excessive stretching. Imagine, then, the impact of relaxin on the nerves at synaptic junctions and you can imagine, as I do, junctions that spread so far apart that the neurotransmitters that should be speedily channeling from one nerve to the other cannot actually reach their end points enough to cause nerve transmission. Now, imagine relaxin in the brain and you can probably see the same problem as I do – relaxin is bad news. Our brain is a giant sponge in part due to the flexibility of neurexin and neuroligin.

Pregnant women sometimes experience brain fog, poor concentration, forgetfulness and absent mindedness – a temporary issue attributed to pregnancy "hormones" as a class. However, it is very likely we could point to relaxin as a major factor in this. What if a person's brain swam endlessly in this hormone due to chrnic infection rather than a few of the 40 weeks of pregnancy, and you should see where I am leading. It is very likely that mental decline as we age has relaxin as a major contributing factor. Senility and Alzheimer's may be an extreme end of what might be a common spectrum of overstretched synaptic junctions.

Recently, my wife mentioned to me that she felt she had suddenly aged a lot in a two month span. Sure enough, her face was filled with relaxin. I cleared this and immediately there was a positive response in the tautness of her skin.

I will stop here a moment and point out two things: first, relaxin is hugely important in pregnancy and therefore is not a bad hormone that should be maligned forever and all time. Secondly, I am an energy practitioner who cannot back up these assertions with any scientific facts – so my energetic finger pointing needs to be taken with a pinch of salt.

There is no "anti-relaxin" on the market that I am aware of – which means that prevention and also fast action when one notices a period of inexplicable, sudden aging, is critical. Follow the calendar at the end of this book for regular anti-parasitic cleanses to help protect yourself against Paragonimus. However, when one experiences a sudden bout of fast aging unexpectedly, such as one's face suddenly seeming very stretched out, a loss of tone in a tissue such as muscle tone, immediately employ the Anti-Parasite Protocol recommended in this book ad hoc as needed.

Lastly, I want to point out a reality of a Chinese medical practitioner versus a Western practitioner. We see there are often multiple paths one can follow that can end with the same Western diagnosis. Earlier, I discussed the importance of DHEA for memory. Here, I am saying taut synaptic junctions are necessary for memory. If something goes awry in either situation, major issues in memory can manifest. Anemia can also cause the same symptoms. Inflammation of the brain can also do this. Which is to say, there is no one gate one must guard to protect the brain – but many. This is why I have written this book, because reading a short magazine article on the subject won't maximally protect you. Instead, you need an array of strategies. Ergo, I have created the calendar in this book. But the calendar is like a wall that has cracks. It will defend against most attacks but it is nevertheless porous. You may employ the Anti-Parasite Protocol one month and the very next month when not on this protocol experience a major, unexpected exposure to parasites. This is life. Which is why the calendar is helpful but you must recognize also when to flexibly apply the protocols in this book. You won't be an expert. You won't do it perfectly. I don't do it perfectly. You do your best. Relieve yourself of the lie that you can do it perfectly. You can't. But at any given moment, you can do the best you can do at that moment. Try your best and see how it plays out. Honest truth, you are still going to age. But in all likelihood you will age with less suffering the more you use the strategies I am sharing.

Key Takeaways:

- Relaxin is a wonderful molecule for labor and a terrible molecule for aging

- At this moment, a parasite called Paragonimus is known to generate this, but it is likely other organisms will be found to produce this over time
- Follow the Anti-Parasite Protocol in this book both at the regular intervals indicated in the calendar in the book but also when you feel you have experienced a sudden acceleration of aging
- Release the expectation you will be perfect at identifying what you need to do and when. Simply, do your best. We are all going to age no matter what we do. The goal is to more often than not intervene preventatively even though we know there is no perfect success rate at stopping the ever advancing clock

Cerebellum, Precognition, And Subtle Muscles

It is most of 2023. I have Covid in January for the first time. My brain is not working right. I am getting through my work day just fine and from the outside, I look the same. Only my wife can tell that words that used to come quickly are missing, needing workarounds. My thinking is muddled. I feel as if I have dropped 20 IQ points. I am still able to plan international trips and travel alone in new localities, so I am functional. But I can tell something is wrong.

I realize this is no joke and that no one is going to solve this issue for me. I tinker on myself, as I am apt to do. I realize my brain is full of isomers of DHEA and that DHEA proper shapes fold differently when comparing visual memory, long term memory, short term memory, lateral thinking, and basic cognition. I clear the isomers and go on a DHEA supplement. I almost immediately feel back to normal...but still not quite normal. I go in and out of periods where I simply cannot find a word. Is this being 51 years old or is this Long Covid or something worse?

It is December, 2023. I am having an episode in which I cannot find a word and it suddenly dawns on me that part of me knows the word I chose was the wrong word. Which means, part of me already knows the right word and knows the word I selected just plain is not it. I realize this part is non-verbal, not quite subconscious but sub-language. I call this the Precognitive Center. I find that it is located in two locations: one is the cerebellum and the other is anterior/superior to the hippocampus, above the lateral fasciculus dorsi, the most important part of the brain for word/noun/proper noun recall.

I'm not done fiddling. I know, for instance, that the cerebellum has shown up time and time again as playing a role in pain and so I realize that the molecules that play a role in pain are supportive of precognition in their proper allotropic shapes. But the more pain you have, the more these molecules are consumed, the more precognition suffers.

This makes sense. But I'm not done. I discover, through happenstance, that enkephalins also support these precognitive brain centers. My system is head to toe riddled with isomers of enkephalins. I clear these and boost the proper shapes only is my brain feeling almost entirely normal, I suddenly feel happy to be at work, a job I originally chose due to my passion for its theory. For three years during Covid, work was a joyless chore with brief flashes of delight. It appears stress and negative experiences boost those isomers, rob life of joy, and when life is dull and stressful, precognition is thrown out the door.

The brain knows what it knows at a level lower than thought. How cool is that? I will answer my rhetorical question. It is very cool. It makes sense to me that this area of precognition is in the more "reptilian" part of our brains, the cerebellum – likely one of the first cerebral areas to develop in multi-cellular organisms. It also makes sense to me that this evolved likely at the same time our neurotransmitter technologies were limited, when we were playing around with only a handful of such molecules. This means we might create "thought" on the back of "pain," because the most basic rule of a body is: "if in pain, escape."

I have spoken of the need for the proper shapes of DHEA for mental function, and I would say this molecule appears to play a gigantic role – but not the only role. Without precognition knowing the coordinates of words/ideas/meaning, thought is errant and absent.

These discoveries speak to the importance of two things: 1. If in pain, get out of pain. Do whatever you can to find a way out of it. You may need surgery as a last resort. You may need Western medicines as a crutch. But I am a practitioner of alternative medicine and I would feel remiss if I did not tell you that you should try everything you can before you get a surgery because surgeries cause pain. Recovery is not a joy ride. Nerves are cut. Wounds must heal. And when it comes to Western medicines that cover up pain effectively, this does not mean those painful isomers aren't still in circulation – they very well likely are. The medicine is likely just hiding your experience of them, but this does not mean they won't continue to negatively impact the Precognitive Center.

Instead, seek physical therapy, osteopathy, chiropractic, craniosacral, homeopathy, naturopathy, myofacial release, Alexander Technique, Feldenkrais, deep tissue massage/rolfing, hypnosis, blue laser, oxygen chambers, and more. There are many, many roads to follow. And you should try them all, if necessary, giving each a solid course of application rather than a "once and it didn't work so I will move on." Of course, what you don't see listed is Chinese medicine and the reason it is not listed above is because I am going to take a moment on my Ted Talk about this.

Chinese medicine is at least 3000 years old but probably goes back at least 6000 years. Ötzi, the 5000 year old man found frozen in the alps between Austria and Italy, of all places, had tattoos at acupuncture points and meridians. By contrast, Western medicine is effectively 200 years old (the modern version of it – not Hippocrates version) and every other technique I mentioned above is not much older. When was the last time you did something more than once or twice when it didn't work? Now imagine having at least 3000 years to abandon a methodology that wasn't serving its core population – a population that ended up covering the entirety of a landmass greater than the United States (most of Asia). Day after day, person after person, this was the primary medicine for millions upon millions of people. You might even say a majority of all humans that have ever lived prior to the modern era were treated by it. I suggest you throw away any prejudices you might have about the unknown. EVERY disease known to man interfaced with Chinese medicine as it was the PRIMARY medicine of all of these people.

I find myself in a funny place as a person innovating with the oldest standardized medicine known to man. I find it endlessly fruitful and, in fact, this book is the byproduct of that fruitful labor. This book is also just the tip of the iceberg of a career of discovery and experimentation. Which is to say, if you throw up your arms and say: "I've done it all" and you have not tried acupuncture, Chinese herbal medicine, or medical Qi Gong then my retort is: "Really? Have you?"

And that was my Ted Talk. Pain conditions are Chinese Medicine 101. There are friendly people around the globe who can assist you even if you are frightened of needles – which I might add, are akin to the mosquito bites you never felt and far removed from the syringes that have a hole at the end of a tube necessary to wound you enough to insert a foreign substance into your body. It sounds far fetched, but just ask anyone who tried acupuncture and they will tell you how astonishing it is to have a needle in their body and not know it has already been inserted.

If in pain; stop the pain. Try every possible option. Do it for the pain and also do it for your brain.

Also, it must be said, for your brain to work maximally, life needs to be fun. Obviously, life is also serious and at times brutal and terrible. But one must fight to maintain joy especially when there are extended periods of darkness. The brain needs this fun as a fuel to keep working optimally. What is fun is different for each person, but it should feel fun. You should be able to think: "that was fun" and feel that is an honest reflection of truth. Doing something you think should be fun but which doesn't actually feel fun isn't actually fun for you at least at that moment in time. So, that does not fit the bill. You must be a seeker of fun and not passive. Find out what life-affirming activity drives your passion and embrace it.

Subtle Muscles

Speaking of subconscious processes or processes below thought, there is another system in the body that is super important and entirely invisible to Western science. Yet, these anatomical components are in every millimeter of your body. These are what I call "Subtle Muscles" or what you can consider "nerve switches." Subtle muscles are "on/off" switches that can maintain their current state for days, weeks, months, and years. They play a role in just about every biological function in your body. Imagine a train track in which there are two paths the train can take and one switch that controls that flow. You can flip the switch and only have one track open for days, months, and years. Or you can flip it back and forth several times a day, according to the needs and activity of the track.

Subtle muscles are akin to quasi muscles/quasi nerves. They have receptors that bond to specific molecules that activate them or inhibit them. Just like all receptors, however, they can be tricked by isomers and chelates as well as isomer chelates and this can cause major problems. For instance, it is not uncommon for isomers to fuse to subtle muscles without being able to release, since our bodies are designed for proper shapes of molecules and usually not adapted to handle wrong shapes. Every tissue and every biological process appears to be impacted by these switches – including areas we focus on with aging: hair follicles, each component of a joint, parts of the brain, memory, bone health, blood vessels, eye strength, and so on. I have spent years mapping out which hormones activate or inhibit which subtle muscles. Aspartate, for instance, is helpful for the Precognitive Center but at super small sizes where they activate subtle muscles here memory.

Which brings up a whole other can of worms. Size. We have been taught that everything in our experience is built on standard units of size and that atoms, for instance, are always one size fits all. However, in nature we see life is full of spectrum and size is always included in such spectra. Others before me postulated that such things as "nano" sized organisms exist and I have confirmed this to be true. For this to be true, it also means their component parts must be made of a different sized spectra of atoms. In my experience, nano is actually quite large when it comes to sizes of scale. What nano sized is to our size, there are similarly smaller sizes to nano and even smaller than that. If you have played with images that are fractal you will better understand what I am saying – that the same atoms with the same electron/proton/neutron numbers exist at many different sizes of scale far smaller than we can perceive even with electron microscopes. This may sound far fetched and it is far and fetched but "far fetched" doesn't mean wrong, it just means it sounds unlikely. Given that we are creatures of perception and we exist within a range of sizes we can perceive, I would not be surprised if anyone said: "no, only what we can perceive is real." That's fine. We do know that even at standard sizes of scale, a proton is made of subatomic particles far smaller than one can perceive. As we go down the rabbit hole of trying to find the one particle that rules them all, we find the hole goes deeper and deeper. It turns out the Higgs Boson isn't the end of the road. It goes deeper.

Anyway, that was a digression from my point: subtle muscles are small and they run on nano or smaller sized hormones and molecules. It is hard to interact with them using current tools at our disposal. It may be that vibrational treatment tools will work better than pharmaceutical ones for these kinds of issues – with homeopathy, rife machines, and other more subtle interventions might be necessary for these subtle muscles. Which is to say, if you are finding you are having aging problems that are not reversing, you might then consider going down this rabbit hole – seeking vibrational interventions for issues that may be too small to address with other means at your immediate disposal.

Key Takeaways:

- Precognition is a self-aware coordinate system that is below thought that mediates consciousness and memory
- This system likely evolved when we evolved pain perception as a mechanism to be aware of pain and then respond appropriately to it cause. Pain works against precognition and diminishes mental function over time
- Stressful, challenging life experiences diminish our joy which is an issue for precognition as it runs on the same molecules that make life feel fun. Make sure to have fun in life to counteract this!
- There are other subtle processes that are below the level of thought that control just about every parcel of our anatomy. If nothing else is helping to resolve a symptom, consider vibrational interventions as this might be the only way to activate this anatomy that is run by molecules that are far tinier than you can imagine

Body Sand & Bulbous Pathways

It is 1976. I am four years old, visiting my great grandmother Julie at the old age home. She is 99. She will go on to live to 107. The entire old age facility smells of urine, stool, and saccarine cleaning supplies as we walk up the stairs. This is the last time I will see my oldest surviving ancestor alive. She is skin and bones and not much filler tissue. She moves slowly like the puppet of an elderly person. Everyone we encounter in the facility is moving slowly in their elder years. Me? I have dry powder and the need to burn fuel. I am bouncing against the walls wanting to get out of there, without any of the wisdom of an older person who realizes this is a once in a lifetime opportunity to see, touch, and embrace someone who predated that century, who lived a life accruing feelings and wisdom. My takeaway at the time: old people are smelly and boring, and they really like blankets. They move awkwardly and slowly. And boy would I like to run around right now. Or laugh. Where is the laughter?

Which brings up a good question which is not "why was there no laughter?" There was no laughter because Great Grandma Julie wasn't a laugher. She was serious and stern, as was the cultural agar from which she grew. The question is: why do the elderly move so slowly? Bonus question: why do they like blankets?

As we grow older, we accumulate sand in our bodies and our blood vessels effectively become sand paper. Am I talking about literal sand like at the beach? No. Dental calculus also known as "tartar" is comprised of whitlockite, hydroxyapatite crystals (the same ones in teeth and bones), octacalcium phosphate, and brushite. Whitlockite is a mineral, another form of calcium phosphate. Octacalcium phosphate is bone and teeth precursor molecule. Brushite is a phosphate mineral. These are rough and tough materials – and you know this to be true if you have ever had a metal appliance in your mouth at full force attempting to dislodge a chunk of molar in order to fix it. Along with these are mineral oxalates such as calcium oxalate. These are all forms of "patholocial crystals" that harm the body. I also find the "bad" type of cholesterol mixed into this crystalline matrix and I feel this is why it has accrued such a nasty reputation.

So far, I have found three pathogens that produce tartar in the body: archaea (a category of infectious organism that is not quite a bacteria and not quite a protozoa), Pseudomonas, and E. Coli. Each of these can be treated as a bacteria, in my experience. Thank goodness infectious diseases abide by body boundaries and only infect one area such as the teeth in this case. Oh, wait? They don't?

There has been grumblings in the scientific community that what happens to the teeth happens to the brain – linking periodontal disease with senility disorders. But I would go one step further and say that any organism will effectively infect anywhere it can given the right set of circumstances. Which means these organisms producing dental plaque can, and I assert they do, produce plaque all over the body.

I have never heard anyone describe what it feels like to be inside an older person's body but as I have entered my 50s, I believe I can now put this to words: if you don't move, you feel fine (to the most part). But if you move, it feels as if while you weren't moving, little invisible gremlins were silently buffying soft tissues with very light/fine sand paper – an impact you only notice when you move (at first). This is gentle sand paper, not the strong stuff. It can buff things to a polish but it won't splinter wood. Which is to say, the sensation is light, at least at first in one's fifties. But given enough time, I could imagine the effect widens and deepens so much that at 99, one might move slowly from the communication of these injuries.

As I cleared these pathological crystals from my body, I noticed another invisible impact. I suddenly felt persistently warmer. These crystals may themselves be cold by nature, but they also reduce the volume of blood in blood vessels, which means less circulating blood and less efficiency in distributing this blood to the outer realms of the human body. Why do the elderly need so many blankets? Because they are full of body sand and it is like sand in a desert at night: shockingly cold.

I recommend following my anti-bacterial protocols according to the calendar at the end of this book as a good preventative against the proliferation of organisms that increase these crystals. I do not feel a person needs to avoid oxalate-rich foods because the oxalates are only a piece of a larger whole. It is thought that a sufficiently high calcium diet will help purge the body of oxalates. But the bigger issue is tartar – a mixture of pathogen toxin aggregated minerals.

Obviously, the tougher question is how does one eradicate complex minerals from the body that to the most part no one has ever heard of? The best answer I have is omega 3s which you can get from fish oils. I also recommend cinnamon, the most Fire Qi food that directly impacts the blood vessels according to Chinese medicine herbal theory.

Bulbous Pathways

While we are on the topic of blood vessels, I want to interject an additional important finding – our blood vessels are tubes that are meant to retain their tubular form. The mineral build up I just discussed will negatively impact the internal open space of blood vessels (known as the "lumen") but the tubular shape of blood vessels can also be compromised internally. Blood vessels are often made of layers of tissue tightly integrated (capillaries are only one cell layer thick and are an exception to this). Just like any tissue, a blood vessel can get an internal infection, not just one on its surface – an infection that can wedge its way in between layers comprising the blood vessel. If the colony swells this interim space, the blood vessel is no longer a smooth tube but can be overstretched and bulbous. Fungal pathogens and yeast like to infect blood vessels, secrete hot hormones that cause edema or build up carbon dioxide and/or methane that generates gas bubbles in between the blood vessel layers. The net effect: a tight, vulnerable pain that is also a very common facet of the aging process. This type of pain demonstrates as sharp pressure mostly felt with use and movement.

The proper approach to ameliorate this issue is to boost oxygen and clear low oxygen ("Damp") environments in the body. However, being hidden internal to the blood vessels themselves, it can be harder to eradicate fungi and yeast that have accumulated in such a particular spot, less accessible to circulation itself (ironically, given that these are conduits for circulation). Therefore, if you suspect this situation, following the anti-fungal protocol for 60 days is necessary. I would recommend bouncing around the different anti-fungal treatment options as you work your way through those 60 days (ie. two weeks on nettle tea then two weeks on pomegranate extract then two weeks on caprylic acid, and keep going that way).

Another Sandy Problem

There is another issue that I am putting last in this chapter, not that it is the least important, but because the problem is practically unsolvable. Our bones are made of a crystal called hydroxyapatite. This is a calcium phosphate crystal that in addition to bones and cartilage, is a primary factor in giving hardness to teeth. These crystals are normally held tightly in bones but there are two factors that cause leaching of these minerals into the soft tissues of the body, where they can accumulate and cause persisting pain. First, osteopenia and osteoporosis are obvious factors in bone loss which will result in the dislodging and redistribution of hydroxyapatite crystals far and wide from the bones. No doubt, most of these crystals are excereted out of the system, but no system is 100% efficient and that includes our excretory systems. Not all of these sharp crystals escape the body, but instead pile up in tissues that are not meant to house pointy minerals. This is particularly problematic in joints and in tissues where compression is necessary for their function such as muscles, tendons, and ligaments.

Secondly, muscles and their tendons appear to absorb local hydroxyapatite crystals when there is an injury. What better way to keep you from using a body part that needs to rest and recover than to fill the injured tissue with sharp minerals that will cause a spike in pain with muscle/tendon compression? This is also a likely factor in the recurrent nature of injuries, as these crystals will not all be cleared from the once injured tissue (again, no system is 100% efficient), creating a local tissue environment more conducive for future/recurring injury.

By the time one reaches the fifties, a fair share of compounding injuries have ensued and osteopenia may be starting, which is why this tends to be the decade when more chronic pains arise that we consider "age related." Many joint replacement surgeries happen in this and the next two decades. At least one reason for this, is that pain that is caused by crystals that are stuck in soft tissues can be strong and unremitting when in motion but usually asymptomatic when stationary.

I wish I had better news about how to eradicate a build up of these crystals in the wrong locations but unfortunately I know of no helpful interventions. Remember, you need to keep your bones, cartilage, and teeth while somehow also clearing the crystals that compose these in errant locations of the body. It is a tall order. The best approach is to to protect one's bones from osteopenia/osteoporosis by eating a full, healthy diet rich in calcium and by engaging in weight bearing exercises such as weight lifting. Prevention is the best approach.

Archaea And Their Destructive Coral

Lastly, there is a category of infectious disease you likely have never heard of your whole entire life that is just as problematic as all of the others I have thus far mentioned called Archaea. These are not bacteria, viruses, fungi, or protozoa, but something unique on the tree of life.

Archaea have only come into my consciousness in the last few years and only in recent months have I discovered that they build up minerals in a diffuse coral-like structure (akin to a buckyball with lots of holes). As the infection grows, the coral expands. Over time, this strong mineral substrate will get to the point that it pulls fibers out of their attachments and permanently breaks apart tissues, effectively destroying the structures in which they have rooted. When attachments are pulled out of their bearings, they almost never re-attach, which means Archaea are increasingly damaging as one ages and their colonies grow ever larger. I believe that Black Walnut is one tool one can use to help clear Archaea and nettle tea is yet another, which means there are tools already within our protocols that can help diminish

Archaea colonies. No unique protocol is needed for these alone. That said, the minerals they leave behind are not cleared by our tools. I imagine there are vibrational medicines that can break down these hard structures so that they cannot expand so destructively over time, but I do not as yet have information to share with you about these in this edition of this book. For problems that involve massive tissue destruction, detachment of tissue attachments, or hard expansions in the body, one should consider the possibility these are being caused by Archaea and their ever expanding coral.

Key Takeaways:

- Teeth tartar is an obvious indicator of a hidden danger – minerals that can build up in the blood vessels and organs due to bacterial pathogen and archaea activity
- Use the anti-bacterial protocols according to the recommended calendar to periodically kill off bacteria to help reduce plaque build up
- Omega 3s and cinnamon are the best available self-care tools to help clear what has already built up in the body
- An indicator of successful plaque removal is more healthy warmth (not to be confused with hot flashes) in your body, as plaque makes one feel cold
- A sharp, vulnerable pain with movement and use may be a sign of Damp Pathogens having worked their way internal between the layers of blood vessels. While this is common, it is a bit harder to clear and requires a more concerted use of the Anti-Fungal Protocol for 60 days to make better headway
- The crystals in bones, cartilage, and teeth can migrate elsewhere during injury or from osteopenia/osteoporosis and re-accumulate in soft tissues. This is a particularly problematic facet of aging as it is very hard to clear these crystals – which means it is essential to eat plenty of calcium and regularly weight train to help protect the bones from bone loss

- If tissues are expanding painfully or attachments of tissues have been torn off their bearings, consider the possibility that Archaea and their mineral "coral" are responsible for this

Pathogen Fatigue Cells; Pathogen Pain Cells; Pathogen Stiffness Cells

It is 1985. I am an eight grader at an Amerks hockey game in Rochester, New York. We are a small city with a feeder team to the National Hockey League. That day, they are giving out awards to local athletes and I am getting an award. I can't remember why. That wasn't the exciting part of the day.

I am running around the stadium and I find myself down some stairs at a dead end alone, but not for long. Suddenly, two kids show up that are larger than me. They seem jovial and in what I interpret as a joking manner, they tell me to give them my wallet. One shows me a knife. The whole thing is such a blur that it takes me decades later to realize they were trying to mug me. I am too young, happy, care free, and perhaps out of my mind to think they were for real. So I say: "no way," and I run out of the stairwell at top speed. At first they chase me, but their smoker teen bodies are no match. I am one hell of an athlete. I ran a five minute mile that year around the middle school track. I am a rocket ship and they are the slow downtown train.

I know enough to be full of adrenaline when I make it to my seat. I am also giddy about how those bozos didn't get me. To my 13 year old brain, that was just a silly episode I didn't take for real. To my 52 year old brain...well, now I am wondering what an idiot I was to be running alone in that stadium. If I was a step slower, how might that have worked out?

Infections come in many different kinds of flavors and often one does not even realize symptoms of disease are from infectious processes. In fact, early in my career I realized most symptoms people have are from pathogen toxins. We very much under-appreciate what 2 billion years on this planet (before the first multi-cellular organisms showed up) has allowed single cellular organisms to develop. We tremendously underestimate pathogens.

Just stop and take a moment to reflect on that number: 2 billion years. Billion with a "b" mind you. The dinosaurs lived for hundreds of millions of years. We have lived for 250,000 as Homo Sapiens, barely a drop in the bucket compared to 2 billion. Barely anything, really. Yet we see ourselves as top of the food chain when in reality to bacteria and viruses, we are totally their food and they can eat us all day in and all day out. They grow in unbelievable abundance, and, to the most part, we don't even realize what is going on. We live in a time of germ theory and yet we totally don't get germs. They are alpha. They live not just at the hottest and coldest locations on this planet, but also in clouds. Yes, clouds. Bacteria have been flying for billions of years longer than humans.

One thing we have failed to recognize about infectious organisms, is that while we have organs that are totally integrated into differentiated tissues that you can pluck out of you and sometimes even replace. Single cellular organisms effectively have organs as well but they are dispersed across their colonies rather than within a single unit or body. We have a spleen that cleans the blood. They have many cells that might work within a colony to do the same thing. And yet, to us one Streptococcus Mutans cell looks like another looks like another looks like another. Meanwhile, they are entirely differentiated. One cell might serve the role of sticking to the body and not letting go. That is its only job. It produces toxins specific to that task. Another cell drills through the surface cells to deepen an infection. That is its only job. A third cell has the job of streaming through circulation in order to find another hospitable location to infect. That is its only job. Infectious organisms even have their own version of white blood cells that will seek out and destroy human white blood cells. That is their only job. We look at infectious organisms and think they are stupid, pathetic little nothings when in fact, they are whole bodies without the filler tissues. When inside a host, they make colony, which is akin to a gland or organ and within that colony. They invite their friends to join them. They differentiate tasks. Some cells only have the role of maintaining the integrity of the colony and that is their only task. So far, I have identified around 20 differentiated types of single cellular cells within a species.

Now, I am not trying to incite you into thinking we need to kill all infectious organisms as if they are intelligent boogiemen out to get us. I am not convinced about the intelligent side of things. I think they are opportunistic, for sure. I think they are pernicious and sinister. But they are also part of an ecosystem. I am not encouraging killing off species of infectious organisms as they serve important roles – such as priming our immune systems, cleansing our systems, and generating resurgence of our internal spaces that need some form of opposition to be inspired to be primed, cleansed, and regenerated. What I am saying, however, is that we have grossly underestimated our opponents.

In the context of aging, this means we should be thinking about infectious disease as playing a role in chronic and aging complaints. I have already written quite a bit about fungal pathogens and their role in this. But I want to highlight differentiated types of infectious organism cells that no one realizes is a thing and so no one is thinking "how can we manage this challenge as we age?"

Pathogen Fatigue Cells

There are differentiated pathogen cells whose singular goal is to slow us down. Some organism grow by making us manic and having us spread disease to everyone in our tribe as quickly as possible whereas others want us to be slow, want people to come to us and spend a lot of time caring for our needs, in order to pass on their colonies. This sounds awful and it is awful but it is also how things work, if you are not wise to the hidden processes. Pathogen Fatigue Cells increase fatigue generating molecules in the body such as isomers of cortisol, isomers of T3, lactic acid, excess sugars, and isomers of caffeine, by way of example. Epstein Barr Virus is a good example of a pathogen that uses this strategy to slow one down. It doesn't have to be a virus, however. Anaerobic bacteria and fungal pathogens are happy to play this game as well. Trust me, live in an environment filled with fungal mycotoxins, and you will be moving at a snail's pace and you will feel toxic and, in medical terms, feel like crud.

Pathogen Pain Cells

There are pathogens that secrete isomers of MMP, alpha synuclein, CPK, Substance P, and other pain generating molecules. These will slow you down and also encourage others to get real close in aiding and assisting you. Yes, these single cellular organisms are truly brilliant strategists. Pathogen Pain Cells make you feel pain and they can be found across all genus and species of infectious disease. The flu is known to cause terrible aches. Fungus and Staphylococcus subspecies of MRSA and MRCONS cause arthritis. Pain slows down thinking and one is less prone to respond to an infection if one can't think straight. Perhaps that is one reason for this attack strategy. I can't tell you why the little invisible fuckers in your index finger joints are causing you pain, I can just tell you that they have specialized cells whose only focus is to induce pain and some organisms have more of these types of differentiated cells than others.

Pathogen Stiffness Cells

This should be self-explanatory as to what these organisms do. They spit out progesterone isomers and testosterone isomers like crazy, leading to stiffness and tightness respectively. If we move less, we breath more exhalations in one space, perhaps filling the air with contagion. We are just a vehicle for further distribution of future colonies.

What To Do With This Knowledge

My goal in sharing these insights is not to wallow in despair that we are being outsmarted by organisms whose average individual cellular life span might be less than 24 hours. Instead, it is to say: never give up and never give in. If you are tired, in pain, stiff, or tight – and you have no surgical or genetic reason for this, then you should not simply sit in these symptoms as a victim, but instead, seek out as many interventions as it takes to resolve these issues. I want to make it abundantly clear, Western doctors and even alternative doctors often make the assumption that old age is symptomatic unto itself. Here, I am saying the symptoms of old age are often the accumulated injustices of living in a body within a microbiole soup, and suffering the wear and tear of decades of daily insults that sometimes can anchor and seem endless. Don't fight old age. That clock is ticking. But fight the symptoms of old age even when everyone around you gives you the insipid message: "it's because you're old." Pardon my proverbial French, but fuck that shit. Don't capitulate to the messaging or the messengers. And I will be honest with you, there are going to be many symptoms that you perhaps are not going to break no matter how hard you try. But some you will. That means less suffering. That is the entire purpose of this book. Suffer less. Enjoy life more.

Key Takeaways:

- Infectious organisms are smarter than you, me, and Einstein. They are older than us, wiser than us, and they can fly in clouds. Can you fly? I didn't think so.
- Follow the calendar at the end of this book, because prevention of disease helps reduce suffering. But know that from day one of your life, you have been in a microbiol soup and from day one what seemed like infections without much strategy have actually been infections with strategies smarter than the smartest person on this planet.
- We can smarten up by <u>not</u> accepting "it's your age" as the reason for fatigue, pain, and stiffness

Mysteries Of The Skin

It is 1971. I am in utero. I literally know nothing.

Ah, the skin. The skin is such a big part of aging because it is what we perceive from the outside and it is the basis of much judgment – self-judgment and also, to be honest, the judgment of others.

As an energy intuitive, I must reflect back to you that the skin, which is the largest organ of the body and, from the outside, seems so prominent, is very very very thin, as tissues go. It is more 2-dimensional in many ways, rather than 3. As a consequence, the skin is the absolute hardest tissue for me to diagnose. It has shared few of its mysteries with me.

Here are some things I know about the skin:

- The stress hormone cortisol causes overstretching of connective tissues, and the more one experiences stress in life, the more likely a person wrinkles from this
- I once had a patient who was having a bout of many actinic keratosis following a hydrocortisone shot and clearing the cortisone seemed to stop this process suggesting areas of persistent high cortisone (likely from pathogens or one's own body rather than from hydrocortisone shots) are probably a factor in spots where skin has darkened and become scaly. I don't have strong conviction in this, however
- Thinning skin is l likely from isomers of pregnenolone building up as this is the same cause of thinning vaginal walls and even thinning GI tract membranes. This suggests the possibility of supplementing with a high quality pregnenolone that is not laced with isomers might help (problem is that manufacturers don't care if their products contain isomers – not even a little bit, which means the possible cure might also fuel the problem)
- Cracked skin is often a sign of poor circulation to the skin
- Lip sores are just as commonly not Herpes related as often as

they are and my recommendation when sores show up is to saturate a cotton ball with hydrogen peroxide and hold it onto the ulcer for 1 minute. If it goes away by the next day, it wasn't Herpes but an infectious pathogen that more often than not causes fever that you just successfully defended yourself against (this includes the internal "skin" of the inside lips/cheeks/and tongue)

- If you look unusually pale, go to the doctor to see if you are anemic as this can cause a host of problems such as fatigue, dizziness, shortness of breath and more that is often qualified as "aging complaints" when in fact it is a disorder than be treated
- Pathogens infect melanocytes which spit out a whole lot of melanin. If I clear the melanin, freckles go away and moles lighten but don't go away. This has no effect on liver spots or actinic keratosis
- Darkening of skin, if not from excess melanin, can sometimes be from too much pregnenolone (often a byproduct of infections)
- Protecting the bones keeps the skin taut. Bone loss is a bigger issue for major skin sagging than cortisol
- Relaxin is a hormone toxin that some organisms produce that will cause massive overstretching of the skin
- In my experience, Botox often contains within it active infectious organisms of Botulinum pathogen and its co-infecting pathogens of Hystolitica Amoeba, and Tinea (likely at super tiny sizes known as "nanos"). Not recommended. These organisms are truly bad news and not worth the cost of smoother looking skin

God, I wish I could tell you more about skin. I really do. Crossing my fingers that version 2 of this book has a giant manifesto on skin. This likely will come as a great disappointment to people since we attribute so much baggage to skin.

[s](Age) Age Backwards

Key Takeaways:

- It is frustrating to admit, but after more than two decades in my field, the skin is an elusive bastard that holds its secrets closer than a paranoid spy. I don’t hate it. I just hate what it is doing to me as I age in my skin without answering all of my endless questions as to why

Mice, Cockroaches, Ants And More Oh My

It is 2003. My wife and are living in Jamaica Plains, Massachusetts. We loved our apartment when we saw it originally, when it was full of the last renter's stuff. However, upon moving in, seeing it in all of its naked glory, we are immediately struck by the fact it is actually a tenement building full of holes the size of fists, broken windows, broken front locks, and more. In later months, when we bring the state inspector in to review the property and he is cited for 19 health code violations he tells the state he fixed all issues only for the inspector to return to find he actually did literally nothing, allowing us a legally, clean way to break our lease, he accuses us of being spoiled suburbanites (my non-spoiled wife is from rural Maine), taking no responsibility for his greedy, repulsiveness. But that's not the point of this story.

This apartment is abundant in life. In order of size: we are graced with fruit flies, grain weevies (moths that eat all your flour and grains leaving their maggots throughout your food), endless mice munching in our room at night, and under our bedroom in the basement, a litter of abandoned kittens. This is a verdant space. It is where we conceive our first child.

This is window of time when heroin has become cheaper than cigarettes, and people are being mugged at gunpoint at the end of our street. So hell yes, we high tailed it back to suburbia as quickly as you could say: "code violations." But we moved in as a twosome and grabbed our next apartment in Newton Corner as a two-and-growing-some.

The older people get, the harder it is to address infestations. In my work with elderly patients, I have found that infestions become a "least of my problems" issue. This is not the case at all. Yes, when joints are failing causing major mobility issues, when eyes are failing causing major limitation of one's visual field, and when it can be hard to mentally compute the many data points life throws at us daily – often intentionally by people who prey upon those who struggle with the cognitive load – it does seem that if something has to give, it probably should be the seemingly harmless critters chewing away at the baseboards. With reduced auditory acuity, it would be easy to sleep through the munching.

Mice and cockroaches are representative of two issues. The first one is external. They are an exposure to infectious diseases because the byproducts of these organisms are not just toxic but contagious. There is a reason we chase mice out of the house. They can carry the plague, typhyus, leptospirosis and more. Cockroaches also carry the plague, E. Coli, Cholera, and more. Cockroaches secrete toxins terrible for the respiratory system and are a common cause of asthma in children. Mouse poo should be considered a biohazard. And while these are small and mouse pee is small, it creates toxic air that often people living in infested spaces for weeks no longer are able to smell and so feel the threat has gone away.

The second issue I have with infestations of any sort is one you might call spiritual in nature. I find that infestations in one's living space are a sign of radioactive isomers building up in the body. This may sound terrible and evoke thoughts about Chernobyl, but it is actually a common byproduct of infectious diseases to be exposed to radioactive isotopes. The flu uses this toxin, by way of example, to generate tremendous heat. These are clearly not isotopes that have a long half life. However, if one has rodents, one likely also has some infectious process currently or had one recently that generated or is generating this kind of furnace level internal heat.

It can be hard to clear infestations especially if one is physically ailing. But this chapter is here to make you take a vow and here it is: "As I age, I vow to never live in an infested space." That's it. That's the vow. You take this vow, and you are grabbing the mantle to always eradicate infestations whenever they arise. And they will. You are vowing to be vigilant.

Imagine for a moment that you are living in a moldy house and the air is completely saturated with mycotoxins. That would be bad news, no? Fatigue will ensue. The body will feel toxic. That is exactly the same problem with air saturated with the toxins of rodents and cockroach urine and excrement. The impacts are highly inflammatory. It is tremendously reducing of mental faculties. This is another reason why the elderly tend not to address these issues – because they are mentally stunned by the toxin load. Vow to always attack infestations as soon as you discover them.

I haven't spoken much about ants, though they are in the title of this chapter. While they are very visible in their infestations, they tend to be quieter and less toxic. But they bite. Spiders and centipedes bite also, but these are white blood cells of your house that will eat other infesting agents. Assuming these are a few random individuals and not a whole infestation unto itself, let those critters stick around where they are unobtrusive as guards against infestation. But go after the ants because they bite more readily and more often if they can. Large carpenter ants are also a sign of water damage to one's house as are termites. Water damage means mold to hunt for and address.

Key Takeaways:

- Vow to clear any infestation of rodents and insects in your house as these are not innocuous and can create toxic air that will cause fatigue and mental decline
- Call in friends, neighbors, and professionals as necessary if you are unable to tackle the issue yourself. Don't wallow in the infestation, as this will be an accelerant to aging

Fermenting In Inflammation

It is 1976. I am four years old. My eight year old eldest sister wants nothing to do with the four year old twerp scamming for attention. But my six year old sister can sometimes be coerced into a little fun. The fun starts with chasing around the house. The mid point of our fun is her running into our parents room and shutting the door, resulting in a tug-of-war on either side of the door handles. The end point of fun was when I slipped and my finger got caught in the door jam as the door crashed closed upon it.

I have no memories of my grandfather Stanley being a robust human as all of my memories are clouded by the Parkinson's he later developed when I was old enough to spend memorable time with him. But a robust Stanley finds me holding my finger moments later in what is a bloody mess for half of the last digit was shorn by the door's bite. What ensues next is a bunch of moments in my memory. First, in the bathroom, the first moment I look down at my finger and realize I have hurt it. Up until that moment, there was no pain but upon the revelation that it was injured – all of the inflammation strikes at once. Second, the car ride to the hospital in which it is obvious to a four year old that the game of "punch bug" was a critical piece of rushing to the emergency room. Third, the doctor at the hospital gives me something putrid to drink followed by the choice: would I like a shot in my arm or my buttocks. Again, four year old thinking: "I need my arm for sports but not my butt." Mistakes were made.

Inflammation is a giant piece of aging. However, this is a short chapter in this book not because the topic is unimportant or inconsequential but because inflammation is a byproduct of the issues I have described in detail in pretty much all of the other chapters. If these other issues are addressed and a calendar of prevention is put into action, then will there be inflammation in your life? Hell, yes there will be, because life is full of shots to the butt, metaphorically speaking. But the overall inflammation in the body will be much reduced compared to what is possible if you follow my advice. Think of each issue I have raised as a potential layer of inflammation and that for each you address, that layer is rendered moot. You are still living a life in a microbiol soup. You are still going to have clutzy moments as a biped living on non-flat surfaces. There are genetic factors that are not raised in this book that are still at play that may factor into cardio-vascular disease or one's rate of bone loss. We do not have perfect bodies and this is not a perfect world for these imperfect bodies, which means I make no promises about the strata of inflammation you personally must wrestle with. However, I definitely believe that you will have much less baseline discomfort if you apply the principles outlined here.

In Chinese medicine, we talk about roots and branches. A symptom is a branch of something deeper: the root cause. Western medicine is a functional medicine that is designed to keep people on their feet and to reduce down time as much as possible and inasmuch, it focuses tremendously on the branches – the crutches that get us through the day. In this and in regards to emergency care, Western medicine is a star above all else. But it is absolute shit for roots. Yes, it can stop each UTI or each vaginitis episode, but does it even try to stop the pattern of UTIs or the pattern of vaginitis that extends over years and decades? Occasionally it does, but more often than not it is focused on triaging the moment. Chinese medicine prides itself on focusing on the root and that means it is slower on the branches but deeper in resolving the pattern. Which is to say, focus on the other chapters in this book as the root for inflammation.

That said, there are plenty of ways to relieve inflammation outside of non-steroidal anti-inflammatories. There is great homeopathy, for instance, such as Arnica. CBD oil to rub on inflamed tissues. Blue laser therapy to reduce inflamed tissues. Saunas are a big hit in my family. Turmeric, ginger, peppermint, licorice, and cumin are all used to reduce inflammation (not together, mind you). You can probably guess what I am going to promote as the best choice of all. Try acupuncture. Try that 3000 year old medicine that has worked day in and day out addressing musculoskeletal pain. Yes, I said Chinese medicine is slower at the branches, but it also can be faster. It depends on the person and the problem. If you are wondering if across all of the landmass of Asia where Chinese medicine was the primary medicine day in and day out, whether the hard toiling laborers who were injured and inflamed got blue laser or homeopathy to address their immediate inflammatory needs? No, they didn't. They took Chinese herbs. They received acupuncture and medical Qi Gong.

Lastly, I will say that if you are experiencing enduring inflammation and you have been told by a doctor that this is just a facet of old age, find another doctor. You should not be inflamed on a chronic basis. Look for new ideas. Be a seeker. I have had tens of thousands of patient visits so far in my career and there have been those I could not help and I didn't ever once tell them it was their old age that was the cause – I referred out. For those in chronic pain, you are on a journey. Sometimes the journey is in stages where you can release layers of inflammation over time rather than everything all at once. The journey may lead to different people with different ideas over time. But don't stop until the journey is over and your body feels much better. I am reminded by a Shakespeare phrase said by Hamlet: "There are more things in heaven and earth, Horatio, Than are dreamt of in your philosophy." So seek more ideas, and broaden your philosophy. From a more recent movie that is almost a Shakespearian tragedy with the homonymous name: "Never Stop Never Stopping." You owe that to yourself. You are deserving of comfort.

Super Tiny Pernicious Factors

It is 1994. I am weeks away from graduating from college. I live in an apartment and it is my night to cook and clean up. A piece of angel hair pasta has hardened at the bottom of the pot. I can't get it to dislodge from the metal, so I have the bright idea to scratch it off with my nail. Suddenly, I am in enormous pain. The thin, hard noodle has injected itself under my nail, surprisingly deeply. It is like a splinter but somehow much, much worse. As I dig at it, the noodle does not pop out but instead crumbles, meaning I am able to excrude only a few bits but the rest of the noodle becomes harder and harder to reach.

Honestly, I am in a sort of panic as I didn't even know this could happen and I have no life wisdom to fall back on. I wiggle a pliers as deep as I can get it. It hurts like a mother fucker to get it in there. I aim for deeper than what can be easily reached. The pain is terrible more now by my own choices and actions than by the original insult. Somehow, magically, when I close the pliers on the noodle, it does not shatter and it does pull out. How could something so small cause me such a huge trauma. I am a 52 year old man reflecting on this episode. I have eaten many meals of angel hair pasta and have cleaned many pots of pasta over the ensuing decades. But, yes, I am a man with pasta trauma.

In Chinese medicine, we have a concept called "Pernicious Factors" which is a slightly different way of describing infectious disease. Pernicious is a great word as it really speaks to the sneaky danger of some microscopic attackers.

I am **not** a homeopathist but I am aware of a theory within homeopathic circles that when you use antibiotics to cure a problem, instead of it going entirely away, the problem clears symptomatically on the surface but actually deepens. Such an issue can then be passed from parent to child in what is known as a "miasm." In my career, I feel I can make sense of this by taking a theory I did not come up with myself around super tiny infectious organisms that are smaller than the normal size scales that we can perceive in petri dishes or with microscopes. Organisms are sometimes found in super tiny sizes called "nanos." From a Western perspective, this is entirely theoretical, but in my work, I have found this to not only be very real, but also important in my daily work to ameliorate people's symptoms. Everything exists in a wide spectrum of sizes, including infectious diseases. Antibiotics can only kill what is similar in size – larger sized organisms – but they cannot kill the super small sizes: nano and, dare I say it, even smaller sizes. When homeopathy says that a pathogen such as Tuberculosis goes deeper, I believe it means that while the large sizes are gone, the sizes that are too small for Western medicines to clear, persist – and can remain in an active, infectious, and yes, pernicious, manner.

Homeopathy has tools for infectious diseases called "nosodes" which are homeopathic remedies made by the energy of the same organisms that are being treated. They even have an emotional model for how people feel and behave that reflects the super small sizes of scale of different infectious organisms that can then be treated via these nosodes. I believe this theory is spot on and I want to bring to your awareness two important nano sized creatures that are common factors in our aging, but are beyond our conscious awareness because they cannot be diagnosed via blood tests, scans, MRIs, or any monitoring devices as they simply are way too small to be detectable.

Tuberculosis is a disease that is thought to be eradicated from most of the planet and yet continues to seemingly spontaneously show up in the worst of human environments such as poorly maintained prisons. Which means, it is not actually gone, just invisible, for all intents and purposes. I have found that TB likes to attack little sacks in our bone marrow where stem cells proliferate and then differentiate into different cell types. As a byproduct of its activities, it produces little protein balls called granuloma that can then build up hard nodules. As we age, hard nodules do appear more regularly in visible locations such as the skin, but it is where we cannot see them that these can be a larger factor – such as in ligaments and tendons at their bone attachments where they can cause pain, at the septum and nasal turbinates where they can induce snoring and sleep apnea. On a personality level, the Tubercolinum condition (as a homeopath would define it) is one in which one feels as if time is running out and lives with a frenetic sense along with a feeling of having missed out on life's opportunities. In many ways, this describes many people in their older decades.

The second pathogen to take note of us Syphilis, which similarly exists in nano sizes and tends to congregate in connective tissues, where this increases stiffness and tightness as an additional contributing factor in the discomforts common in an aging body. According to homeopathy, the Sypholinum personality reflects high anxiety around health issues with fear of dying playing a large role. A loss of hope around recovering is also a big component of this. Extreme pain and loss of memory are also part of this personality profile. Again, these are very common aging symptoms.

I am not a homeopathist. I do know that homeopaths would recommend homeopathic medicines to address these issues, but a professional with knowledge about dosage and who can adjust any intervention according to the needs of the patient is tremendously recommended. Which is to say, I do not recommend self-treatment. Homeopathy also has a host of other diagnosis around other infectious pathogens, but these are the two that I want to bring to your attention.

I have not included the clearing of these pathogens in any protocol, as there are no great self-care options outside of nosodes. You cannot, for instance, take colloidal silver or goldenseal to clear pathogens these small. However, I do highly recommend that each reader seeks input from a homeopathist about these emotions if they are presenting.

Key Takeaways:

- Some problems are from infectious organisms way too small for medicines and herbs to eradicate, called “nanos”
- Some diseases people think are eradicated or think cannot be their issue due to lack of sexual promiscuity, are actually passed on at super tiny sizes from ancestors – homeopaths believe these are passed parent to child in what are known as “miasms”
- Sudden increase in the fear of dying or a fear of missing out in life should precipitate a visit to a homeopath

Age Related Pathogens

It is 2004. I am holding my newborn baby who literally just arrived on planet moments earlier. Our eyes lock and we are making sense of our new reality. I had just been crying like a baby out of happiness and she had just been crying like a baby for having just inhaled muconium on her eventful exit from the birth canal. Yet, this is a moment of stillness. We are sizing each other up. I ask her if her middle name is Esther, my running favorite, or Edith. She makes gas pains at "Esther." It is our first decision as a budding family. Edith it is.

I realize as I hold her that my life just changed and that it never goes back in the opposite direction.

Life is not rife with moments like these that are one way trips into a different mode of being – but when they arrive, they are usually quite intense and often jarring. Sometimes they are wonderful such as my story above, but often they are traumatic one way streets.

As a seeming non-sequetor, but that I will tie right back up – our genes are made up of sections that are called Introns and Exons. Exons consist of genes that produce the proteins that make up our cells and tissues, hormones, steroids, cell receptors, peptides, and more. Introns for many years were called "junk DNA" as they were not known to code proteins. In recent years, some additional uses have been identified by Introns, but I believe there are other factors here not yet determined by Western science.

Everyone knows that viruses inject their DNA into cells and this is a strategy of attack. I have found that other organisms that are not viruses also can infiltrate human cells as well. It is also clear the infectious organisms are regularly bonding their DNA with other organisms. A famous example of this is the many variants of Sars-Cov-2, also known as Covid 19. While it is thought that mutations cause its many variants, in reality these organisms swap DNA very eagerly with other organisms, resulting in fast changes in their sites of attack, toxins they produce, and ability to evade the immune system. Which is to say that it should come as no surprise to anyone that human DNA has infectious organism DNA within it.

It is my belief that organisms can spontaneously infect the body via their DNA hidden in Introns already in our DNA at birth and that this happens under various circumstances. A common factor is the exposure to certain toxins. It was common during Covid for people to develop shingles – a painful neurological syndrome caused by Herpes Zoster. It did this by releasing toxins that awoke dormant Herpes in the body.

Not only are pathogens essentially hiding in "DNA form" chronically within our chromatin (our own genetic material), they pop out regularly when it suits their purposes – which are twofold: to spread as far and wide to as many hosts as possible and to deepen within any single one host inside the body to a point where the infection can never be fully eradicated. It appears different pathogens detect environments that are best suited for reinfection not only based on toxins in circulation but also by the age of the host. By way of example, Epstein Barr Virus (EBV) goes around the community every year like a cold – which means people at every age are hit by this infection regularly. And yet the syndrome called "Mononucleosis" – a super massive assault of EBV almost always strikes young people around 18 to 22 years old. It is very age specific.

The same thing is invisibly happening as we get older and is a major factor in periods of sudden aging. There are infectious organisms that are very very old that I call "Primordial Pathogens." These are unusually small (nanos) and also are tremendously destructive to tissues, essentially tearing them apart (think bone loss that shows up as osteoporosis). Unlike parasites and many pathogens that essentially live somewhat symbiotically with the host, Primordial Pathogens don't mind killing the host as a byproduct of their massive destructive force. Major destruction of certain systems can lead to this such as destruction of the heart, blood vessels, kidneys, the pancreas, and the brain. Which is to say, a huge part of the aging process is likely hiding in our DNA at birth and has nothing to do with the number of telomeres capping our genes.

Not all Age Related Pathogens are Primordial Pathogens and as wantonly destructive. But what they all share is the same fundamental property – they are emerging out of our "own" DNA and as a consequence, the infection is like an ongoing waterfall of pathogenesis. Once these start their resurgence, no amount of self-care can stop the root which is hiding in our very own chromosomes, which means all care is palliative – which basically described most of Western medicine geriatric care.

As the entire class of Primordial Pathogens are "nanos" (which mean nano-sized infectious organisms), has not yet been supported by Western science, it should come as no surprise that there are no specific Latin names for specific types of Primordial Pathogens as yet. In my work today, I have only a short list of known non-Primordial Pathogens that I have specifically identified so far, though I am certain I will identify far more in the next few years. EBV is one. Neissaria Meningitidis, a bacterial pathogen that causes extreme neurological pain is another. Clostridium Perfringens, a cause of bone loss is a third. I also suspect certain yeasts are also hiding in this manner.

Peptides are molecules that activate specific genes, acting essentially like switches that either keep genes expressing themselves on an ongoing basis or inhibit genes from expressing themselves at all. For Age Related Pathogens to activate and become an enduring waterfall of pathogen expression throughout one's aging process, which I believe is the case, this must be mediated by the right peptides connecting to the right locations in the DNA, switching on the DNA that was previously dormant. Therefore, there must be certain peptides that increase at different aspects of our aging process that are the trigger for fast aging events and also enduring aging over decades.

I introduce this theory as a novel theory of aging and so there are absolutely no herbs or supplements that one might turn to. Perhaps the "Blue Zones" where people age slower might reflect dietary sources of peptides that are protective or a diet that might reduce peptides that are otherwise dangerous. It is clear that people who exercise regularly age slower. People who meditate age slower. People who eat more vegetables and less meat age slower. This implies that these are inhibitory of the bad peptides. Which is to say, the same rules around diet and exercise you have heard before still apply. Meanwhile, I will keep doing research and perhaps over the next years/decades I will have better self-care recommendations for you that work within this very important domain.

Key Takeaways:

- Our DNA has Introns that hold from birth the DNA of infectious organisms that can spontaneously infect under the right circumstances (with aging itself often presenting those right circumstances)
- Peptides connect to our DNA and act like switches to turn on specific genes or to inhibit them
- Peptides therefore are likely the main factors in awakening dormant infections hiding in our DNA
- Toxins from other organisms can activate these dormant pathogens
- Peptides that build up as we age are also likely a factor in awakening these dormant pathogens
- Sudden aging events (aging quickly) are almost assuredly a sign that pathogens are surging out of the DNA
- High vegetable diets, daily exercise, and meditation likely reduce dangerous peptides that activate these pathogens

A Host Of Diseases

It is 1981. My grandmother passes away from cardiovascular disease at 65 years old as a lifelong smoker. It is 1984. My grandfather dies of a broken heart, never recovering from the loss of his life long love. It is 1996. My grandfather dies of advanced Parkinson's. It is 2004. My grandmother dies of advanced dementia, something akin to Alzheimer's.

People die from a lot of varied issues. Yes, the general rule is cardiovascular disease is going to kill most people due to habituated eating of very fatty foods and not exercising sufficiently, but the reality is that in the end, everyone dies differently. Over my career, I have had patients die of heart attacks, alcoholism, Alzheimer's, cancer, the sequeliae of cancer surgeries run amok, gangrene post Covid (a rare situation), and, in particular, pneumonia. I have also had a fair share of very elderly patients who circled the toilet a few rotations in a very terrible, inescapable spiral that very likely started with severe depression from immobility, loss of function, and feelings of abandonment. It is clear that the survivors of other people's loss struggle tremendously in our culture. Isolating at any age, this is terribly isolating for the elderly, who tend **not** to live in mixed age homes in the United States and can end up feeling very alone.

The facts are that while young people are universally healthy and glowy, as people age, they tend to follow all kinds of craggly branches of unique forms of biological doom and gloom. Many might go down one large limb of cardiovascular disease, or another large limb of metastasis, but even this can end with many different little branches that look unique from one another person to person. Ten out of ten babies all look pretty much the same. Ten out of ten elderly patients, each have their own array of diagnosis.

My goal in this book was never to write about specific diseases such as Alzheimer's, Parkinson's, ALS, cancers of all sorts, or more.

Why? There are simply too many chapters in that kind of book. That book is an encyclopedia. What I will say is that there are what appears tipping points for most people where they are doing just fine but then something gets a hook in them that pulls them into a darker space and that this tends to especially be a danger in one's 80s.

In Chinese medicine, we say all diseases stem from one's emotions. I am entering my 25th year in this medicine and I have not been disabused of this idea – though everything is clouded widely by the body experiencing very real symptoms. The Western world calls this "psychosomatic," as if it were a disease as opposed to the actual way that life works. It is all somatic and it is also all emotional.

I therefore believe that much of the diseases experienced by the elderly are truly diseases of the heart – traumas never processed, childhood emotional scars that have grown over decades, grief especially as one's friends and family suffer and die, festering anger, a desire to not see something impending or fear of facing some brutal truth. It doesn't help that cognitively and intellectually humans age in an arc that I metaphorically say follows school cycles. We start in elementary school then progress through middle school, then high school, and, for some, college and graduate school. For much of our lives we live at the peak of this intellectual capacity, but eventually the curve reverses and intellectually and emotionally we revert backwards – high school, then middle school, then elementary school, and then we end the cycle. Imagine the capacity of a very aged person and you can see at the far range, it is not far different from a toddler's capacity. If you can see that, I hope you can get my analogy. If we are lucky to live long enough, we see the whole arc. But this also means that as we hit the later decades, we are no longer as sophisticated in our strategies for addressing the intense emotions that dictate our health. There is more time and less emotional capacity, yet no less emotion – in fact, an even greater accumulation of feelings that span decades.

I am not going to talk about a host of diseases in this book. Instead, I am going to talk about one: the disease of drowning in intense, unresolved emotions. This is the disease of the elderly. It is the disease to take most seriously and to afford great energy into combating. Funny then that it is so unrecognized in our world of tremendously over-prescribed medicines and great ignoring of the wrinkled folk's feelings. According to Chinese medicine, it isn't Alzheimer's you need to be frightened of, it is simply this: a heart unexamined. It isn't cancer. It is this. It isn't a meteor hitting the planet precisely where you are standing. It is you not working on your shit while you have the intellectual capacity to still do it.

Everyone has trauma. Everyone. I have lived a particularly easy, simple life. I don't carry too much trauma. But I have trauma. I have PTSD. I have a bridge phobia, as you know, and I have trauma from that. I have shared with you only one of many similar stories. I also have experienced heart break. I have friends who rejected me whom I thought would be my brothers in arms forever. I have unresolved childhood feelings that I do actually work through periodically, but they are there and real – yes, so many decades after I left my nuclear family of origin, those feelings are still present. It doesn't take long to pick at those scabs and feel real pain. If they are in me, they are in you. What can you do for your long term health? Get a great therapist. Find someone you can talk to and process your life. Fight isolation. Find community. Even as people suffer and die, find more people, and especially younger people. Fight age discrimination.

In terms of therapists, I am agnostic as to the type, but I advocate that you find someone who talks rather than prescribes. If you need prescriptions, get prescriptions. But also find someone who can find the roots of your feelings through conversation and not just work on the branches by numbing the feelings.

Does this mean you will avoid diseases? In Chinese medicine, we would think that it does. I cannot stand here and assert that you definitely will. However, the oldest canon of Chinese medicine, the thousands of years old text that still teaches practitioners to this day, certainly believes this is the case. Will you get a disease and a diagnosis as you age? Assuredly. But perhaps you can make your list a short one rather than a grocery list of ICD 10 codes (Western medicine insurance codes) simply by learning more about yourself and the context of your life's experience.

Key Takeaways:

- Your emotions are more dangerous than all of these terrible diseases you have heard about your whole life
- Everyone has trauma. These are hidden minefields just waiting to show up one day as some disease. So root this out of your spirit
- Age with a therapist. Even if you have to pay for community and conversation, it is a pathway to fend of isolation and feelings of abandonment

Opioid Receptors And Other Shockingly Important Things

It is early July 1989. I am 17 years old. I am sitting in a circle on a flat mountain top in Israel overlooking the city of Jericho. Flash back two hours ago, we were in the desert and everyone on the bus was told to drink their full water cantina as one can dehydrate quickly in the "negev." I fail to compute the fact that my cantina is twice the size of everyone else's. Flash forward an hour. We are hot from an hour sitting in the desert listening to a history lesson. We are told that everyone should fill up their cantinas with water and then drink it all to avoid dehydration. My initial failure is now secretly exponential. Everyone else drank the volume of two cantinas whereas I drank the equivalent of four.

I am sitting in that circle overlooking Jerico. The other teenageres around me are strangers to me that I met two days earlier. Our circle is matched by not just one more circle but perhaps twenty to thirty more circles of people receiving a history lesson about Jericho. Receptors in my bladder that normally never fire are now firing strongly. They are saying to my autonomic nervous system: dude, you're totally screwed. You have to pee now or you are going to pass out. I am literally hopping where I am sitting, shaking my body, doing everything I can do to not think about my bladder as it expands, expands, expands.

Finally, my teacher takes notice and asks me what the heck is going on. I tell him I have to find a bathroom badly. He shares that there are no bathrooms here. He tells me to go urinate over the mountain cliff. Did I mention I am 17 years old surrounded by hundreds of strangers? I am caught between the humiliation of peeing myself, passing out and peeing myself, or peeing in front of hundreds of strangers. I am perspiring in a country where one normally does not even know one is perspiring because the dryness evaporates it so quickly. But I can feel it this time. Beads of perspiration.

I am well aware that Israel is embroiled in the second Antifada, with overboiling anger and violence between Palestinians and Israelis. I am terrified by the thought that perhaps an insult of peeing towards Jericho might elicit some response from the fine citizens of the city far below. Nevertheless, I am without options. I am standing on a cliff overlooking Jericho. There are hundreds of strangers behind me. It takes the gears in my urinary tract some time to process that I am allowing this to happen but finally, I am relieving myself. It continues and continues and continues. The teacher stops his lecture to point out that, wow did I actually really have to go. I am still going. This turns out to be the longest pee of my life – four cantina equivalents worth, all bottled up. When I am done, my system is very confused as to whether I am humiliated or relieved. Both, it turns out.

There are all kinds of receptors in our bodies. We tend to think of the more basic set of pain and pressure receptors but there are innumerable ones that one does not think about. For instance, caffeine only stimulates us if we have receptors that connect with it. We only have receptors that connect with caffeine because our bodies actually make endogenous caffeine that is part of the wakefulness cycle of our circadian rhythms. Some people have more of these receptors than others and find exogenouos caffeine (ie. from coffee) too overstimulating. Others have few of these receptors, are very groggy in the morning, and indulge in cup after cup happy to indulge in as much exogenous caffeine as possible every single day. Caffeine makes us happy and alert. It therefore attaches to receptors that activate these faculties.

Takes this logic out to what you might consider an extreme, and you have to ask yourself why recreational drugs have the impact they have in us? Cannibis has the same root as the Canninaboid System, a neurological system that reduces pain, increases happiness, and reduces stress. The names are similar because they are related. Molecules in marijuana attach to these receptors and activate them. Why do we have these receptors? Because we have are own endogenous molecules that also reduce pain, increase happiness, and reduce stress. Some people have a lot of these receptors and appear happy and low stress all of the time and there are those with few of these receptors who are regularly struggling with pain, a negative mood, and a high sensitivity to stress. Similarly, our bodies make our own endogenous opioids, which makes us susceptible to the use of opioids. For thousands of years, Chinese medicine has utilized morphine to reduce cough, as this opioid system inhibits the lungs while also increasing positive feelings.

In much of Asia and Africa, there are large populations of people addicted to the Areca nut also known as the Betel nut. These nuts contain arecoline, a molecule that is very similar to opioids and caffeine – they are stimulating, reduce pain, and increase a buzz. The nut and its method of consumption are full of carcinogens, making the people addicted to this nut very endangered. The nut only works because we have arecoline receptors and that means we also make endogenous arecoline.

You can see a pattern here – a lot of the factors that make us feel good are addictive. In Chinese medicine, we say too much of a good thing is not a good thing and that is the truth when it comes to the exogenous forms of these molecules for which we have receptors designed to handle a small amount of endogenous versions of these same substances. Our bodies adapt to too much by making more receptors and thereby needing more stimulation to have the same level of activation that previously was possible with less of the activating molecules. This is called "tolerance," and it is a very bad thing because tolerance is addiction. Remember, when I said that people with too few receptors for the cannabinoid system have less tolerance for stress, a more negative mood, and more pain? This is also true not just if there are too few receptors but if there is too little of the molecule that stimulates those receptors. And when you build up tolerance, you suddenly need more and more of the molecules to keep those receptors activated or else that same array of negatives ensue.

As we age, we are prone to problems on both sides of the equation: too few working receptors or not enough of the substrate that is needed to activate them. Obviously, the solution is not to become addicted to recreational drugs. However, the solution for many is to become reliant on Western medicines that have pretty much a similar benefit, but that are better controlled so that there is less likelihood of a dangerous overstimulation – an overdose – and death.

Add to this, a big reduction in stimulation, activity, adrenaline, and joyful events and you can see why so many of the elderly appear to age depressed, angry, sour, and in pain. The problems here are too much for a single person to navigate. You need a team of healers to be able to figure out for you whether you are low in receptors or low in feel good molecules that stimulat them.

It is common for the elderly to self-medicate with alcohol for its mind and body numbing capacity. Alcohol is one of the worst drugs available to the public. Think of it more as an anesthetic than a cure to the problem. It is a depressant, which means that it slows down the system and is inhibitory. It chews up the liver. It is easy to become addicted to it without realizing it because a little "toddy" at night quickly becomes a necessary sleep aid, even though the alcohol itself will wake you up in the middle of the night.

So, where does that leave us? Should we all be chewing betel nuts or snorting cocaine? I certainly don't think so. Should we all be medicating with Western medicine and stimulate our systems with more refined, medical approved stimulants? Maybe? At least this comes with a physician keeping tabs on our well-being, which is a plus that does not come from buying heroine from a friendly neighborhood pusher.

Here is the bottom line: we do have receptors for these molecules and we do have a physical and emotional need to have endogenous molecules that stimulate us in the way highly addictive molecules do to excess. We need to keep these systems primed but not overcharged by exogenous versions that cause addiction. The absolute best way to do this is to embrace stimulation – embrace travel. These are all Fire Qi molecules that increase joy, passion, and love. We have a certain number of alternative options with cinnamon, chocolate, coffee, and black/green tea. Beer is a Fire Qi food but as I said it can be easily abused and is highly caloric, so is not on my recommended list. Finally, exercise is the number one thing to do that stimulates all of these receptors. I am not a fan of marathon running on how it negatively impacts the feet and knees, but there is a "runner's high" for a reason – the more one exercises with vigor, the more "positivity" receptors that are activated. One should age with movement. Dance, especially.

Key Takeaways:

- Our bodies can be addicted to substances that reduce pain, increase positivity, and reduce stress because we make our own endogenous (human made) versions of these same molecules and have receptors that seek to attach to these molecules
- Addiction is the result of having receptors for these molecules and the negative impact of overstimulating these systems, resulting in tolerance
- The elderly can have too few receptors or too little endogenous molecules, resulting in an increase in pain, anger, sadness, and higher levels of stress
- Keep your receptors toned with healthy mechanisms of vigorous exercise, Fire Qi foods, travel, and stimulation
- Don't drink alcohol to fall asleep as you will quickly become addicted. Plus, it worsens insomnia over time

Western Medicine Preventative Care I Recommend

I am a practitioner of alternative medicine and for pretty much all things, I lean in that direction. However, I do believe in Western medicine as an important piece of regular healthcare, especially when it is pulled apart from the insurance companies and pharmaceutical companies that inject capitalism into the domain of medicine, which I argue should be protected from capitalism and seen instead as a natural born human right. These forces are a rot that even its own practitioners will admit has sickened allopathic care. And yet the only cure for this is political – whether nationalized healthcare, price controls on medicines, or protections from lawsuit abuse. Given this rot, it can be hard to divide what is truly helpful regular self-care for aging gracefully and what is corporate greed that has foisted itself on a process that could be cleaner and more patient-centered but just plain isn't.

The vaccine schedule is one such place of confusion. When Rotavirus kills 100 people a year in first world nations, should it be included in the required vaccines for children to attend school? How about poliovirus, which could cause life long paralysis? Should that be in the vaccine schedule? One seems pretty darn important and the other seems like a corporate interest more than a human interest – can you figure out which one is which? Of course you can.

There are many people in alternative circles who think all vaccines are terrible. And yet Polio is a good counter argument. Smallpox is another. The alternative circles often have a principle of "purity" that vaccines violate in that they are often filled with activators, stabilizers, and preservatives – sometimes even mercury and other heavy metals. Most of this is junk that just makes it easier to preserve vaccines to be used over time for multiple patients before these high priced items go bad in the fridge. I am not apologizing for the use of these chemicals but I can at least see the logic behind them. Meanwhile, what is not considered is that pathogens produce toxins that can include heavy metals, paralytics, poisons of their own making, blood vessel cloggers, fatigue generators and more. Which is to say, to avoid an infection is also very protective of the body of a host of terrible impurities that no one who cares about their internal purity wants in his or her system.

I therefore hang out in the uncomfortable middle when it comes to vaccines and feel that there are some that people absolutely need and there are those that we should wonder if perverse incentives are fueling their marketing and use. I therefore recommend various vaccines and the one that I recommend the most will surprise many people. I absolutely 1000% recommend that everyone gets a Tetanus shot every 5 to 10 years. My patients who do not do so invariably suffer neurological problems as they age as well as disorders that include tightening of body parts (sometimes but not always involving the jaw). In every cut from metal, I find Clostridium Tetanii, the pathogen that is prevented with the vaccine. EVERY SINGLE CUT. Which is to say, its ubiquity cannot be ignored. I don't know about you, but I am a clutz, and I cut myself periodically. I most definitely cut myself multiple times a year with metal.

As for other vaccines, I recommend the Polio shot, Mumps, and Measles. If your work will bring you in contact with blood, I recommend Hepatitis B. These are hugely important for preventative purposes. Recently, I have been finding Neissaria Meningitidis to be a very terrible organism for causing chronic pain and therefore recommend the Meningococcal vaccine as well to help prevent neurological pain disorders. I also think that vaccines that stop highly infectious, deadly pandemics are worthy as well. I am not saying all other vaccines are bad or all others are driven by pharmaceutical greed or insurance company money saving, or the desire to keep corporate employees in the office rather than recovering at home. I just think that the others are not as essential as these.

If you go to the dentist and are told every time that you take impeccable care of your teeth and gums, do you really need to go every 6 months? For decades, I went every 2 years and was told the same thing every time: "you look great – come back in 6 months." But recently, the tartar has become much more prevalent and harder to clear, indicating a change in my circumstances. I am now going more regularly because being adaptive to change is ideal and because the same tartar on teeth builds up in the blood vessels as arteriosclerosis, in my opinion, which means it is important to keep this under control as best as one can.

Are colonoscopies necessary? They will detect approximately 150,000 cancers a year in the United States. Colon cancer is the 2nd largest killer when it comes to cancer deaths. But here's the thing – the prep and process is absolutely terrible. 15 million colonoscopies are performed a year with less than 1% of cancers found across this population. What makes this a tough call is that there are stool tests that are not invasive at all and require 15 minutes of time rather than days of preparation. Are these perfect? No. But, these stool tests are already highly accurate and only improving over time. It is therefore my feeling that unless there is a pre-existing condition (ie. Crohn's disease, family history, genetic predispositions), why wouldn't a stool test suffice, with a follow up colonoscopy as necessary? Yes, there are risks – but all facets of life carry risks.

My physician father feels statins should be in the water supply but I am skeptical of Western medicine's focus on cholesterol. Cholesterol is the main hormone to convert into pregnenolone which converts into the top most important hormones you know by heart without being in the domain of medicine: ie. estrogens, progesterones, cortisol, testosterones, etc. A medicine that reduces cholesterol may negatively impact the body far and wide. C-reactive protein, homocystein, and lipoproteins correlate with heart attacks far more than cholesterol. I am not telling you to not take a prescribed statin – perhaps your diet or genetics necessitates it. But if you exercise regularly, eat healthy, and have a healthy BMI, should you be overly concerned about slightly elevated numbers? I personally don't think so.

I think baseline EKGs are a good idea. Preventative action can be helpful with heart issues picked up early.

There can be helpful data in blood tests – but really only if you take years of patterns into account more so than one item being elevated on one test here or there. The exception to this of course being if that an indicator means there is an active, acute problem that needs immediate remediation. However, blood tests are akin to photographs and can only tell 2-dimensional stories. Oftentimes, they are swayed by recent infections that people didn't even know they had. That said, knowing one's A1C blood sugar score is also very informative. Knowing iron/ferritin/hemoglobin levels is important as low level anemia even at marginal levels on blood tests can actually be highly problematic symptomatically (a rare occasion where I feel blood tests are actually under-valued). Which is to say, I do believe blood tests can be helpful. But what I feel most doctors miss is that these are useless out of the context of a person's diet, exercise, and history of viral infections within the last 4 weeks – which are three things doctors don't spend enough time evaluating.

If you have blood tests with information outside of normal ranges, take more blood tests over time. Watch to see if the pattern gets better or worsens.

Lastly, I want to say the following about Western medicines. I recommend treating these like Chinese herbal formulas. Take them for a specific, delimited time period and then re-evaluate whether or not you still need them. Western doctors have a tendency to prescribe life long medications as standard practice of care – again, without also recommending lifestyle changes that might effectuate improvement in the underlying conditions. What if every medicine that was prescribed was re-evaluated every 6 months or every year not with the question of "should I increase the dosage?" but with the question: "Is this still necessary for my ongoing well being?" Don't go off prescribed medications without discussing this with your prescribing physicians as this can be dangerous.

In terms of aging, the reason I advocate this is that tools become blunt when they are over-utilized but can remain sharp if they are used in thoughtful, distinct, potentiated ways. If an anti-depressant helped once but was thoughtfully reduced and stopped when no longer needed, it makes sense that that the same pharmaceutical tool will be helpful again in the future and, when utilized again, will have known side effects and also a known ability to help. Instead, the standard of care is often to put a person on a medicine and wait for it to stop working, then move to another class of medicine that will need to be tolerated, yet has unknown interactive impacts in the patients' unique system. I advocate that you work with your doctors to use medicines when you need them, itemize what work, reduce what you can when you can, and return to those that worked again should that once again be necessary in the future. Important caveat – I am not a doctor and I am not trained in Western pharmaceutical medicines. I cannot imagine how many doctors hate me now for advocating for more conversations about medicines. Simple rule: if what I just wrote doesn't make sense, ignore it. But just maybe it makes a whole lot of common sense. Meanwhile, eat healthy and exercise, work on your root constitution, and see how far basic self care gets you in between epochs in which you need pharmaceutical crutches to get by.

Alternative Medicine: Is It Necessary?

Just as I have skepticism about some Western preventative care, I have similar thoughts about alternative care as well. Not everything "alternative" is golden. There are plenty of supplements and shiny, brand new methodologies that are snake oil. Aloe, a fantastic herb, is the coldest food you could possibly eat energetically, and therefore it is absolutely **not** the cure for every disease known to man. It helps where it helps, but it is sold like it is a panacea.

Vitamins and minerals are often not necessary for people if they eat enough vegetables. However, there are times when taking these make sense – such as a diagnosis that would benefit from supplementation (ie. osteopenia/osteoporosis), or after an illness as part of one's recovery. I feel the same way about probiotics. If you eat a wide array of foods, you should not need these. However, if you have taken a lot of antibiotics, this might be a time to consider it, though I believe this is only introducing monoculture to your flora rather than a wide rainforest of species.

There are also plenty of the latest and greatest, newest, and most exciting healing methods being thrown at people who are open to alternative medicine. I recommend healthy skepticism. It is important to know the difference between something that makes you feel good versus something that does good for you. Maybe what you are doing fills you up with endorphins but doesn't turn the dial at all for long term benefits. If you try new things, evaluate if you feel there was more than 24 hours improvement, as anything 24 hours or less is likely the placebo effect of a short term boost of feel good hormones.

Key Takeaways:

- Some Western preventive care is good for you and you should take very seriously but the most important preventative care, diet and exercise, are completely off your doctor's agenda, which is a genuine shame
- Capitalism should not be in medicine. It is a rot
- Consider re-evaluating medicines with your prescribing doctors every 6 to 12 months so that you can age with tools that are effective for your unique physiology that are not allowed to become blunt by excessive use over time
- Not all alternative medicines are worth your money. If your improvement is 24 hours or less, it is the placebo effect, not actually healing you

The Reverse-Aging Calendar

The title of this chapter is simultaneously tongue-in-cheek as well as a legitimate goal. I say this because there is no real clock. There is no objective metric. Though some people here and there profess to having a system to identify your body's age compared to your calendar age, there is no universally codified metric where you can measure apples to apples. At the same time, there are subjective metrics such as (by way of example):

- Feeling more vital
- Having more stamina
- Being more active
- Experiencing less pain
- Feeling subjectively as if aging is going slowly
- Feeling "More Thrive-y"

My goal is for you to be able to see the items in this list improve or stay constant in a good range for you. And the goal for this calendar, is to provide you with a systematized, date-based protocol that you can follow to best reach this objective.

I do need to say that this protocol will not work for everyone, especially for those who are aged and haven't had the good fortune of receiving this book in earlier decades of life, resulting in deeply rooted, chronic infections. The deeper an infection, the harder it is to see improvements with these protocols and the more you should seek a professional healer's help in getting you back on pace where this book will then prove fruitful for you.

Our calendar focuses on periodically throughout the year clearing fungal pathogens, anaerobic pathogens, bacterial pathogens, and viral pathogens, strengthening the eyes, and eating a diet one month a year that helps to clean out the blood vessel walls and improve circulation. However, when it comes to bacteria and viruses, these are incredibly volatile and variable. Approximately every three weeks a new virus and/or bacteria starts to bloom in the community especially during indoor times of the year (for most people in the Northern hemisphere this is late October to early May). The protocols here are for more chronic infections and not the acutely attacking rat-tat-tat of daily living. For new, acute infections, see the Protocols and apply them ad hoc as needed and don't wait for a date to show up on the calendar before you counter-attack an acute infection.

In this calendar, you will see a differentiation between Northern Hemisphere (Northern) versus the Southern Hemisphere (Southern). In this schedule, fungal and anaerobic pathogens are cleared four times a year, every three months. Viral and bacterial pathogens are treated less often. But as I just said, treat these whenever they hit as needed with our protocols.

REVERSE AGING CALENDAR

January

Northern Protocol: Anti-Parasite.

Northern Protocol: Increase Fire Qi Foods (dark chocolate, cinnamon, coffee, black tea, green tea) to benefit mood. Take 1000mg of cinnamon once a day this month.

Southern Protocol: Anti-Viral

February

Northern Protocol: Anti-Viral

Northern Protocol: Increase Fire Qi Foods (dark chocolate, cinnamon, coffee, black tea, green tea) to benefit mood. If you live under grey clouds most of this month, take 5000 IU of vitamin D unless otherwise directed by your doctor.

Southern Protocol: Anti-Fungal. Anti-Anaerobe. Include protocols for yeast. Mid January to third week of February is the beginning of the Late Summer in Chinese medicine, a different season than Summer. Dampness abounds. Fungal pathogens are Damp Pathogens. The second and third weeks of September, drink 2 cups of nettle tea a day to clear Dampness.

<u>**March**</u>
Northern Protocol: Anti-Fungal. Anti-Anaerobe. Include protocols for yeast. If you live under grey clouds most of this month, take 5000 IU of vitamin D unless otherwise directed by your doctor.
Southern Protocol: Anti-Parasitic

<u>**April**</u>
Northern Protocol: Anti-Bacterial. Take omega 3s daily this month.
Southern Protocol: Anti-Bacterial

<u>**May**</u>
Northern Protocol: Take A Break – eat a vegan diet (or at least vegetarian)
Southern Protocol: Anti-Fungal. Anti-Anaerobe. We have just finished Autumn and tree molds need to be cleared. Take elderberry or echinacea or astragulus once a day this month to rev up the immune system. If you live under grey clouds most of this month, take 5000 IU of vitamin D unless otherwise directed by your doctor.

<u>**June**</u>
Northern Protocol: Anti-Fungal. Anti-Anaerobe.
Southern Protocol: Take a break – no protocol
Southern Protocol: Increase Fire Qi Foods (dark chocolate, cinnamon, coffee, black tea, green tea) to benefit mood. If you live under grey clouds most of this month, take 5000 IU of vitamin D unless otherwise directed by your doctor.

<u>**July**</u>
Northern Protocol: Anti-Parasitic
Northern Protocol: Reduce Fire Qi Foods (dark chocolate and cinnamon) and eat more fruits, especially watermelon
Southern Protocol: Anti-Viral
Southern Protocol: Increase Fire Qi Foods (dark chocolate, cinnamon, coffee, black tea, green tea) to benefit mood. If you live under grey clouds most of this month, take 5000 IU of vitamin D unless otherwise directed by your doctor. Take 1000mg of cinnamon once a day this month.

August
Northern Protocol: Anti-Viral. Take elderberry or echinacea or astragulus once a day this month to rev up the immune system.
Southern Protocol: Anti-Fungal. Anti-Anaerobe. Include protocols for yeast. If you live under grey clouds most of this month, take 5000 IU of vitamin D unless otherwise directed by your doctor.

September
Northern Protocol: Anti-Fungal. Anti-Anaerobe. Include protocols for yeast. Mid August to the third week of September is the beginning of Late Summer in Chinese medicine, a different season than Summer. Dampness abounds. Fungal pathogens are Damp Pathogens. The second and third weeks of September, drink 2 cups of nettle tea a day for to clear Dampness.
Southern Protocol: Anti-Parasitic

October
Northern Protocol: Anti-Bacterial
Southern Protocol: Anti-Bacterial. Take omega 3s daily this month.

November
Northern Protocol: Take a break – no protocol
Southern Protocol: Anti-Fungal. Anti-Anaerobe.

December
Northern Protocol: Anti-Fungal. Anti-Anaerobe. We have just finished Autumn and tree molds have stopped rotting on leaves especially with snow or a Winter frost. In the last week of December, kill yeast buildup from the holiday's sweets and treats with caprylic acid. If you live under grey clouds most of this month, take 5000 IU of vitamin D unless otherwise directed by your doctor.
Southern Protocol: Take A Break – eat a vegan diet (or at least vegetarian)
Southern Protocol: Reduce Fire Qi Foods and eat more fruits, especially melons. In the last week of December, kill yeast buildup from the holiday's sweets and treats with caprylic acid.

	Northern Hemisphere	Southern Hemisphere
January	Parasites	Viral
February	Viral	Fungal/Anaerobe/Yeast
March	Fungi/Anaercbe/Yeast	Parasites
March (last week)	Eye Exercises	Eye Exercises
April	Bacterial	Bacterial
May	Eat Vegan/Vegetarian	Fungal/Anaerobe
June	Fungal/Anaerobe	break
June (last week)	Eye Exercises	Eye Exercises
July	Parasites	Viral
August	Viral	Fungal/Anaerobe/Yeast
September	Fungi/Anaerobe/Yeast	Parasites
September (last week)	Eye Exercises	Eye Exercises
October	Bacterial	Bacterial
November	break	Fungal/Anaerobe

December	Fungal/Anaerobe	Eat Vegan/Vegetarian
December (last week)	Eye Exercises, Clear Yeast	Eye Exercises, Clear Yeast

Build Your "Age-Well" Healthcare Team

Western medicine is at its strongest when its practitioners work together. The bad news is that this is rare – more likely during emergencies in the hospital than day-to-day in the real world. When they work as a team, they spot things early and react more quickly which is perhaps why Western medicine is the absolute best when it comes to medical emergencies. Daily life is not moment-by-moment acute medical emergencies and so this is where the ties that bind Western allopathic care quickly become threadbare. It is common for one doctor to not know what another prescribed – for one doctor to not know what another diagnosed – and for multiple doctors to not have enough cumulative information patched together to make a complex diagnosis for a problem that is multi-factorial. If you have ever had to seek out a Rheumatologist or have had undiagnosed chronic Lyme disease, you will absolutely get what I am saying.

Unless something dramatically shifts in Western medical care, I think it is fair to say this is the situation – Western care is an army of walled gardens – and it is not going to change. If it isn't going to change, *you* have to change in order to age optimally. One way you can do this is to force your doctors to work together. I cannot imagine how many physicians who just read that line just cringed – because the last thing a tired, overworked, stressed out doctor wants to do is to organically on their own time and through their own power create these lines of connection with other practitioners. For a single patient, this isn't such a big deal, but for every patient to make these kinds of requests across a wide array of practitioners and specialists would be a wild web of chaos. I can see why doctors simply won't do this.

Instead, I suggest you create a team of alternative healthcare practitioners. Alternative medicine is usually not as overburdened by patient numbers and by after-hour responsibilities. Sometimes they have to do insurance billing, which eats up tremendous time, but sometimes they opt out of insurance and have even more bandwidth. You want practitioners who don't look at each other as competitors but as a healthcare team of independent operators who can each contribute a piece of the puzzle that is you and who can integrate information coming from different people to inform how they move forward for your care.

Obviously, Western doctors are critical infrastructure when it comes to one's medical care and what they add is often critical information. The diagnostic tools they have are objective and often clear cut. But if these practitioners are the outer perimeter planets in your orbit, you want inner planets who see you more often and who can be lighter on their feet in terms of adjusting to your more immediate needs based on the external input of other trained professionals.

You will absolutely find there are plenty of alternative medicine practitioners who are not open to this. There are plenty who want a sense of control or who have ego limitations that won't allow them to take in other people's opinions but their own. These are people I recommend that you fire from your healthcare team and replace with others who are less egoically driven. Instead, look for open minded people who simply have your well-being in mind and who can set their egos aside for a moment to consider the opinion of others. Daily, I hear other practitioners' opinions on my patients and sometimes I reject them based on my experience but just as often I run with their ideas to see if I agree. These can be absolutely critically important moments in my patients' care, as I only have one brain, one point of perspective, one set of conversations with patients, one educational path that I have experienced, and I cannot see the whole picture even though I try my best at every turn. That said, I am also not the greatest healthcare team member because my practice has been so successful that I often have much after work hour patient responsibilities – making my time, energy, and focus far more limited when it comes to communicating with other healthcare practitioners. There is a sweet middle – a cadre of practitioners with just the right amount of work/life balance who can really integrate with others in a fantastic manner. Find these people and make them "My Healthcare Team."

The absolute best healer on your healthcare team is a seeker who is curious who also has these attributes of open mindedness. Such a person will take the puzzle of you and really try to figure you out. If you can find a great integrator of information such as this, you have won the Healthcare Olympics. But even if you end up with an array of people doing their best within their limitations, you are so better off than you would be navigating your aging process alone. Find a great team! That is your homework.

Types of practitioners to consider adding to your team include:

- Acupuncturists and Chinese herbalists (as often as recommended)
- Osteopaths or Chiropractors (as often as needed)
- Naturopaths (activating during acute health crisis)
- Massage therapists (as often as needed)
- Oxygen Chamber owners (according to the schedule in this book)
- Homeopaths and/or Kinesthetic Testing Practitioners (at the onset of a new major health crisis)
- Therapists to help resolve slow smoldering emotional traumas (and then whenever there are high stress life challenges)

Types of Western care practitioners you should also see regularly in a wider orbit:

- Primary care physicians (annual check ups and also whenever needed for acute situations)
- Dentists (at least every 2 years minimum if all is going well, but every 6 months as the situation requires – notably **not** getting x-rays every visit)
- Eye doctors (according to your needs or their recommended schedule)
- Cardiologists (at least every 5 years and whenever concerns might arise)
- Specialists that have been brought in for pre-existing conditions (as needed)
- Nutritionists (to make sure your diet promotes dense and strong bones)

Key Takeaways:

- You won't likely find a collaborative team of Western medical providers but instead Western doctors are effectively a set of walled gardens walled off from each other. You should not expect that to change
- Instead, form your own team of alternative medicine healthcare practitioners of people who can put their egos aside and listen to the opinions of others, as this team will help you during times of crisis (ie. during the sequelae that follows a Western medical emergency) and can also help put together more complex diagnostic puzzles that any one single practitioner might miss

Conclusion

Yes, aging can be a pearl of embarrassing misfortunes that invariably involve suffering, loss of youthful pizzazz, and a serious challenge to one's dignity. But also "yes," you absolutely ***can*** age better.

Rule number 1: Fight aging. Absolutely never accept the collective trance behind the all too common refrain: "it's just aging." Reject it every single time.

The goal is maximum homeostasis. This book provides council on how to maintain this as best as I am able. But don't stop with me. Collect your healthcare team with whom you can navigate these choppy waters together. Don't try to do this alone. A captain wouldn't sail at night without a compass or stars for guidance.

Do not accept the dark emotions that can come with this process. Wrestle angels and demons, work on trauma, seek higher ground, and protect your emotions as these guide your physiological circumstance in many ways.

Fight fight fight infections. We live in a microbial soup and we even have pathogens in the Introns of our own DNA that emerge as we hit aging milestones. Fight every infection with gusto. As a habitual exercise, look at every new aging circumstance as infectious in origin.

None of us fail to go deeply into the final ocean. But when you do, I hope you feel the journey was eased by (s)age advice and much encouragement.

Age well, my friend.

Alphabetical Index

www.ingramcontent.com/pod-product-compliance
Lightning Source LLC
LaVergne TN
LVHW052259200926
848481LV00002B/410
9798992870008